Basics of
HUMAN GENETICS

Second Edition

Basics of
HUMAN GENETICS

Second Edition

Versha Katira
MBBS, MS (Anatomy), FIAMS (Genetics)

Former
Professor and Head, Harsaran Dass Dental College, Ghaziabad

Vice-Principal, Professor and Head, Department of Anatomy
Santosh Medical College, Ghaziabad

Professor, Department of Anatomy
Christian Medical College, Ludhiana, Punjab

Associate Professor and Head, Department of Anatomy
LLRM Medical College, Meerut, Uttar Pradesh

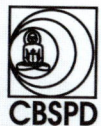

CBSPD

CBS Publishers & Distributors Pvt Ltd

New Delhi • Bengaluru • Chennai • Kochi • Kolkata • Lucknow • Mumbai
Hyderabad • Jharkhand • Nagpur • Patna • Pune • Uttarakhand

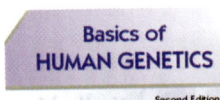

Basics of
HUMAN GENETICS

Second Edition

ISBN: 978-93-86310-68-2

Second Edition: 2017
Reprint: 2022, 2025
First Edition: 2014

Published by Satish Kumar Jain and produced by Varun Jain for

CBS Publishers & Distributors Pvt Ltd

4819/XI Prahlad Street, 24 Ansari Road, Daryaganj, New Delhi 110 002, India.
Ph: 23289259, 23266838   Website: www.cbspd.com
                                e-mail: delhi@cbspd.com

Corporate Office: 204 FIE, Industrial Area, Patparganj, Delhi 110 092
Ph: 011-4934 4934 Fax: 011-4934 4935   e-mail: publishing@cbspd.com; publicity@cbspd.com

Branches

- **Bengaluru:** Seema House 2975, 17th Cross, KR Road, Banasankari 2nd Stage, Bengaluru560 070, Karnataka, India
  Ph: +91-80-26771678/79   Fax: +91-80-26771680   e-mail: bangalore@cbspd.com
- **Chennai:** 18/8B, Subbarayan Street, Shenoy Nagar, Chennai 600 030, Tamil Nadu, India
  Ph: +91-44-42032115, 26681266   Fax: +91-44-42032115   e-mail: chennai@cbspd.com
- **Kochi:** 42/1325, 36, Power House Road, Opposite KSEB, Kochi 682 018, Kerala, India
  Ph: +91-484-4059061-67   Fax: +91-484-4059065   e-mail: kochi@cbspd.com
- **Kolkata:** 147, Hind Ceramics Compound, 1st Floor, Nilgunj Road, Belghoria, Kolkata 700056, West Bengal, India
  Ph: +91-33-25633055/56   e-mail: kolkata@cbspd.com
- **Lucknow:** Basement, Khushnuma Complex, 7-Meerabai Marg (behind Jawahar Bhawan), Lucknow 226 001, Uttar Pradesh, India
  Ph: +91-522-4000032   e-mail: tiwari.lucknow@cbspd.com
- **Mumbai:** PWD Shed, Gala No. 25/26, Ramchandra Bhatt Marg, Next to JJ Hospital Gate No. 2, Opp Union Bank of India, Noorbaug, Mumbai 400 009, Maharashtra, India
  Ph: +91-22-66661880/89   e-mail: mumbai@cbspd.com

Representatives

• Hyderabad	0-9885175004	• Jharkhand	0-9811541605	• Nagpur	0-8692091830
• Patna	0-9334159340	• Pune	0-9664372571	• Uttarakhand	0-9716462459

Printed at Goyal Offset, Kundli, Haryana, India

Preface to the Second Edition

I would like to thank my colleagues and students, whose constant endeavor inspired me to write this second comprehensive edition. Based on appropriate suggestions, this edition includes detailed explanation of the basics of genetics with illustrations, flowchart, etc. A new chapter on common genetic disorders is supplemented with profound illustrations. Descriptive and objective questions have been given at the end of each chapter to improvise learning.

As the science of genetics is metamorphosed into interesting facts, and becomes an integral part of medical education, I have tried to explain the basic underlying facts in detail. The book correlates the basics of genetics with clinical aspects of common genetic disorders in a lucid and easy-to-understand manner. Various branches of cytogenetics, biochemical and molecular genetics are explained extensively for better understanding. The clinical aspects have been outlined in tabular form, wherever necessary. Hopefully, this assertive effort will surely help undergraduate and postgraduate medical, dental and paramedical students in imbibing the elements of human genetics.

Versha Katira

Preface to the First Edition

I have been encouraged by aspiring students and colleagues to make an attempt diligently to unfold this interesting and fascinating branch of medical sciences. Recently, genetics has become an essential and integral part of medical education, both at undergraduate as well as postgraduate levels. It is still undergoing metamorphosis and gaining momentum rapidly for its expansion.

Thus, a suitable, comprehensive and compact textbook of human genetics is unavoidable. Most of the students find the subject too difficult to grasp and are not able to correlate the underlying principles for most of the genetic disorders. Thus, I have tried to correlate the basics of genetics with clinical aspects of some common genetic disorders in a simplified and understandable language and thus making the subject interesting.

Various branches of the subject, e.g. cytogenetics, biochemical genetics, molecular genetics, etc. have been dealt extensively for better understanding while the clinical aspects have been briefly outlined in tabulated forms, wherever required.

I sincerely hope and wish that the first attempt will serve a useful and meaningful purpose in the field of medicine.

Versha Katira

Acknowledgements

I am extremely grateful to all the colleagues throughout my career in different colleges for giving the full support and criticism on the first edition. Special thanks to Dr Molly Paul, Christian Medical College, Ludhiana, where I completed the first edition of this book. I owe my special thanks to Dr (Mrs) Krishna Garg for her inspiration in writing the second edition to this book.

I am extremely thankful to the editorial team at CBS Publishers & Distributors, New Delhi, and specially, Mr Y N Arjuna, Sr Vice President, Publishing, Editorial and Publicity, for his constant encouragement.

I will gratefully acknowledge every comment and suggestions from teachers and students leading to improvements in the text as well as the illustrations.

Versha Katira

Contents

Historical Aspects

INTRODUCTION

Human genetics is the branch of medical sciences, which deals with the study of hereditary materials passing from one generation to another. The study leads to a better understanding of the way by which these hereditary materials develop into physical characters under the influence of intrinsic as well as extrinsic environmental factors. In other words, the science deals with the transmission of physical, mental and biochemical characteristics from parents to their offsprings. The science also reasons out as to why an offspring will not be the exact replica of their parents. The tendency on the part of offsprings to reproduce parental features is known as *heredity*. The science of heredity is the youngest branch of all medical sciences. During the last six or seven decades, a phenomenal growth of this science has occurred and thus opened up the biological thoughts for better understanding of some of the problems of life as far as the health of future generations is concerned.

Till the beginning of seventeenth century, the knowledge of reproduction, heredity and development was merely speculative. However, about 6000 years back, the Babylons had prepared stone tablets to indicate the pedigrees of several generations of horses. The Chinese, before the Christian era, improved on varieties of rice by hybridization. Early plant and animal breeders improved the varieties without being aware of the underlying principles involved. It was only in the later part of 17th century, with the invention of microscope, and its effective use, the necessary observations, and experiments, a number of theories and laws were established to explain the mechanisms of heredity.

In 1632, Nehemiah Grew, an English plant anatomist, described the reproductive parts of plant and thus made the experimental plant hybridization possible.

In 1672, Regnier de Graff, a Dutch surgeon, observed the presence of watery fluid around the ovum in ovaries of females named after him as graafian follicle.

In 1675, Antony van Leeuwenhoek, a Dutch lens grinder, reported about tailed swimming bodies in the seminal fluid of animals including men, seen under the microscope. He named the bodies as *animalcules* and thought that they contain the hereditary material that passes from parents to the offsprings. During the same period, another Dutch microscopist, Jan Swammerdam, claimed to observe the miniature form of man in the head of sperm and named it as *homunculus*, thus giving the concept of 'theory of preformation'. However, at a later stage the theory was negativated by discoveries which proved the importance of both sperm and ovum for transmitting the hereditary material.

From 1838-39, the 'cell theory' was established by Schwann and Schleiden. In 1868, Charles Darwin used the cell theory as the basis to explain the mechanism of inheritance giving the *theory of evolution and pangenesis*. The *theory of evolution* postulated that variations in each individual of a given species after multiplication are the result of recombination and mutation. The *theory of pangenesis* stated that every cell of a living organism produces minute hereditary particles called *pangens* or *gemmules* which reach the reproductive organs via blood stream to form gametes.

August Weismann (1834-1914), the planner of modern genetics, formulated the concept of continuity of germplasma.

Later, this was explained by Samuel Butler (1835-1902) with the statements, "The hen is merely the egg's way of producing another egg". Bateson in 1906 was the first person to use the term 'genetics' derived from Greek word 'gene' meaning 'to become.' In 1909, the term 'gene' was coined by Johannsen for hereditary materials and in 1911, the terms phenotype and genotype were introduced.

Naudin in 1862 formulated the fundamentals of heredity as follows.

i. Repeated hybridization in a race leads to the acquisition of parental characteristics.

ii. The potentialities of both the parents are present together in a hybrid.

The work of an Austrian monk, Gregor Mendel (1822-84) on plants in the year 1865 made him the 'Father of Genetics', as he laid down the foundation of the science of genetics.

The observation of Gregor Mendel in 1869, after the scientific experiments on garden peas (*Lathyrus odoratus*), led him to conclude the reasons for the transmission of characters from one generation to another. He suggested that there are two factors responsible for one character, and these two factors in 1906 were named as genes or the units of inheritance. Mendel also observed that for each gene there is an alternative form present at the same site of homologous chromosome of an individual. A pair of contrasting genes was called an *allelic pair* or *allelomorph*. He also recognised that there are two types of genes, the dominant and recessive. All his work remained unnoticed and unpublished till the end of 18th century. Although, his untiring work led to the formulation of principles of heredity known as 'Mendelian laws'.

MENDELIAN FIRST LAW OF SEGREGATION AND PRINCIPLE OF UNIT INHERITANCE

This law states that the trait or character is always expressed by a pair of factors or genes (alleles) as a unit, originally derived from each parent. Only one member of this pair of genes is found in the gamete, i.e. the two genes always *segregate* during meiosis of gametogenesis. The blending of traits determined by such pairs of genes in offsprings does not occur, as the alleles retain their identity and thus pass unchanged from one generation to another irrespective of their expression in any generation, i.e. the character of parents as a *unit* may not appear in first generation but may appear quite unchanged in later generations.

MENDELIAN SECOND LAW OF INDEPENDENT ASSORTMENT AND PRINCIPLE OF DOMINANCE

This law states that inheritance of one gene of a pair (allele) is unaffected by the inheritance of other gene of same pair. Thus, members of different alleles assort at random and independent of each other. It also states that, of the gene pairs in an individual for contrasting characters, only one gene usually expresses itself and the other is latent. The former gene is named as dominant and the latter recessive. The dominant gene can always express, irrespective of whether it is paired with a dominant or recessive gene, but recessive gene can express only when paired with another recessive one.

The Mendelian work published by Brunn in 1866 in *Transactions of Natural History Society,* remained an obscure publication. It was rediscovered by following three different biologists separately:

i. Hugo de Vries, Professor of Botany, University of Amsterdam, Holland.

ii. Von Tschermak Seysenegg, an assistant in the agricultural experimental station of Esslingen near Vienna, Austria.

iii. Correns, a botanist at the University of Tubingen, Germany.

Thus, genetics started as a separate science not from Mendel's own paper, but from papers that rediscovered his work. In 1903, Sutten and Bovary postulated yet another theory independently known as *Chromosome Theory of Inheritance.* The theory stated that the chromosomes are the carriers of hereditary factors or genes and the behaviour of the chromosomes at the time of cell division provides the cytological basis for Mendel's law of inheritance. Human genetics during the 18th and 19th century prior to Mendel's work was known and reported by simple patterns of inheritance without any proper scientific understanding. The obvious innerited characters, like albinism and polydactyly, were studied by Maupertuis of France in 18th century and Haemophilia was described in a family by Otto from New Hamsphire in 1803. By 1875, the human genetics had grown to such an extent that Galton made a distinction between the effects of environment and heredity and thus making the study of human genetics possible quantitatively in addition to qualitative analysis, thus initiating the polygene inheritance for some of the inherited traits.

In 1888, Waldeyer introduced the term 'chromosome'. Till the beginning of 20th century, human genetics remained in its infancy in the form of tracing the pedigrees and effects of consanguineous marriages. The actual breakthrough has been brought about by a series of research workers afterwards independently. Garrod in 1902-08 was the first to report about the concept of biochemical genetics and it was elaborated by Beadle and Tatum, who gave the hypothesis of *one gene and one enzyme*. In 1900, Landsteiner after discovering the blood group ABO, initiated the study of genetics of blood groups, similarly population genetics started by formulation of a law by Hardy, a mathematician at Cambridge University and Weinberg, a German ophthalmologist known as Hardy–Weinberg law.

Since the last five or six decades the human genetics has grown to a tremendous amount with some of the significant events as follows.

In 1902, McClung identified the sex chromosomes in grasshopper.

In 1916, Bridges started the science of cytogenetics by proving that genes are linearly arranged on the DNA strand of chromosomes in a particular sequence. In 1927, Muller proved that exposure to X-rays, ultraviolet rays, gamma and cosmic rays, etc. and some drugs increases the mutation rate of genetic material by many folds. In 1946, he received the Nobel Prize for this discovery. In 1933, Morgan proposed the function of chromosomes in transmission of heredity.

The genes, situated on the same chromosomes were transmitted together and not by independent assortment. He was awarded Nobel Prize for his work on the nature of gene.

In 1930, Karl Landsteiner received Nobel Prize for his work on blood groups and immunology.

In 1949, Barr and Bertman were the first to demonstrate the sex chromatin in neuron of a female cat.

In 1952, Gerty Cori and Carl Cori demonstrated the first specific enzyme defect an inborn error of metabolism, i.e.

deficiency of glucose-6-phosphatase as one of the glycogen storage diseases.

In 1953, Jervis detected deficiency of phenylalanine hydroxylase in phenylketonurea (PKU). Same year, Watson, Crick and Willkins discovered double helix structure of DNA molecule.

In 1954, Allison clarified the suggestion of Ford and Haldane, about the role of infectious diseases in influencing the genetic constitution of men, by his study of the relationship of malaria and the gene for sickle haemoglobin. In 1956, the human chromosome number was established independently by Tijo and Levan on one hand and Ford and Hamerton on other, to be 46 and not 48.

In 1957, Ingram gave the role played by a gene in determining the amino acid sequence of a protein by his study on normal and sickle cell haemoglobin of men. In 1958, Nobel Prize was awarded to Joshua Leaderberg for his work on sexual recombination in bacteria, and George Wells Beadle and Edward Lawrie Tatum for their contribution in the biochemical genetics. In 1959, Arthur Kornberg and Severo Ochoa, received the Nobel prize for their work on the chemsitry of DNA. In 1959, Lejeune and his colleague for the first time observed a congenital anamoly—Down's syndrome in man providing the basis of chromosomal abberation. In the same year, Nowell and Hungerford were the first to identify the specific chromosomal abberation associated with cancer—chronic myeloid leukaemia.

It was in 1961, MF Lyon gave the hypothesis that in females normally one X-chromosome is inactivated during early developmental period. In 1961, James Watson, Francis Crick and Maurice Wilkins received Nobel Prize for elaborating the structure of DNA. In 1965, RNA was used to achieve protein synthesis in a test tube, thus genetic code was cracked. Francis Jacob, Andre Wolf and Jacques Monod received Nobel Prize in 1965 for finding the genetic control of enzyme synthesis in virus. Hargobind Khorana, an Indian scientist along with Marshall Nirenberg and Robert Holley, shared the Nobel Prize in 1968 for perfecting the test tube protein synthesis of a known sequence of nucleotide as a gene and thus determining the sequence of amino acids in a protein.

In 1970, Hamilton Smith and Daniel Nathens used a new class of restriction enzymes named as chemical scissors to slice and separate the DNA molecules and received Nobel Prize in 1977.

In 1972, Paul Berg in collaboration with other workers combined the DNA from two viruses and called the technique as recombinant DNA.

In 1973, Stanley Cohen and Herbert Boyer inserted recombinant DNA into a host bacteria to reproduce or clone the foreign DNA, leading to beginning of genetic engineering. In 1975, Temin and David Baltimore, were awarded Nobel Prize for challenging the central dogma which hitherto denied the possibility of cytoplasmic RNA directing nuclear DNA synthesis.

In 1977, Genetech, one of the first company for genetic engineering, embarked on the biosynthesis of important drugs by recombinant DNA methods. In the same year independently Federick Sanger and Walter Gilbert discovered techniques for the rapid sequencing or reading of the order of nucleotides in DNA molecules. In 1978, sickle cell anaemia was diagnosed before birth of an infant by analysis of its DNA.

In 1982, human insulin was produced by recombinant DNA.

In 1983, Nobel Prize was given to Barbara McClintock for her discovery that genes can move from one spot to another on chromosome of plant and change future generations of plants. She thus gave the concept of *jumping genes.*

In 1984, the Nobel Prize was given to Niels Jerne, Cesar Milstein and George Kohler for giving the concept of "monoclonal antibodies".

HISTORY OF GENETICS

1866	Mendel's paper published: Units of inheritance in pairs; dominance and recessiveness; equal segregation; independent assortment. These ideas are not recognized for 34 years.
1869	DNA (first called *nuclein*) is identified by Friedrich Miescher as an acidic substance found in cell nuclei. The significance of DNA is not appreciated for over 70 years.

1900	Mendel's experiments from 1866, rediscovered and confirmed by three separate researchers (one Dutch, one German, one Austrian). A British man (William Bateson), soon translated Mendel's paper into English and champions the study of heredity in England.
1902	Human disease is first attributed to genetic causes (*inborn errors of metabolism*). (Sir Archibald Garrod–alkaptonuria).
1902	The chromosome theory of heredity is proposed by Sutton. Boveri recognizes that individual chromosomes are different from one another, but he doesn't make a connection to Mendelian principles. Nevertheless, Boveri is given co-credit by friend EB Wilson (Sutton's supervisor) for proposing the chromosome theory of inheritance.
1905	The word *genetics* is coined by William Bateson.
1905	Some genes are linked and do not show independent assortment, as seen by Bateson and Punnett.
1903-09	First experiments on quantitative traits in broad beans by Wilhelm Johanssen and wheat by Herman Nilsson-Ehle.
1910-11	The chromosome theory of heredity is confirmed in studies of fly eye color inheritance by TH Morgan and colleagues.
1913	First ever linkage map created by a Columbian undergraduate, Alfred Sturtevant (working with TH Morgan).
1910's-30's	The eugenics movement is popular, fueling racist sentiment and leading to involuntary sterilization laws.
1925-27	H Muller shows that X-rays induce mutations in a dose-dependent fashion.
1928	Some component of heat-killed virulent bacteria can *transform* a non-virulent strain to become virulent, as shown by Fred Griffith. This sets the stage for work done in 1944.
1931	Genetic recombination is caused by a physical exchange of chromosomal pieces, as shown in corn by Harriet Creighton and Barbara McClintock.
1941	One gene encodes one protein, as described by Beadle and Tatum.
1944	DNA is the molecule that mediates heredity, as shown in Pneumococcus transformation experiments by Avery, MacLeod, and McCarty. Most people were skeptical of these findings until 1952.
1946	Genetic material can be transferred laterally between bacterial cells, as shown by Lederberg and Tatum.
1950	In DNA, there are equal amounts of A and T, and equal

amounts of C and G, as shown by Erwin Chargaff. However, the A+T to C+G ratio can differ between organisms.

1952   DNA is the molecule that mediates heredity, as shown in bacteriophage labeling experiments by Alfred Hershey and Martha Chase. This confirmation of the 1944 results really convinced everyone.

1953   DNA is in the shape of a double helix with antiparallel nucleotide chains and specific base pairing. This was deduced by Watson and Crick, who used Rosalind Franklin's data provided by Maurice Wilkins.

1958   DNA replication is semi-conservative, as shown by Meselson and Stahl using equilibrium density gradient centrifugation.

1959   Messenger RNA is the intermediate between DNA and protein.

1966   The genetic code is cracked by a number of researchers (including Nirenberg, Matthaei, Leder, and Khorana) using RNA homopolymer and heteropolymer experiments as well as tRNA labeling experiments.

1970   The first restriction enzyme is purified by Hamilton Smith.

1972-73   Recombinant DNA is first constructed by Cohen and Boyer.

1977   DNA sequencing technology is developed by Fred Sanger.

1986   PCR is developed by Kary Mullis.

1990   Genome projects begun. The yeast genome is complete in 1996, and the C elegans genome is done in 1998.

1990   DNA microarrays are invented by Pat Brown and colleagues.

1990   DNA fingerprinting, gene therapy, and genetically modified foods come onto the scene.

1995   Automated sequencing technology allows genome projects to accelerate.

1996   The first cloning of a mammal (Dolly 'the sheep') is performed by Ian Wilmut and colleagues, Roslin institute in Scotland.

2000   The Drosophila genome is completed. The Arabidopsis genome is completed. The human genome is reported to be completed.

2001   The sequence of the human genome is released, and the post-genomic era officially begins.

2009   Controversies continue over human and animal cloning, research on stem cells, and genetic modification of crops.

SELECTED BOOKS ON HISTORICAL FIGURES/EVENTS IN GENETICS

Overviews/chronologies	Examinations of particular people or experiments
Mendel's Legacy: The Origins of Classical Genetics by Elof Axel Carlson	*The Monk in the Garden* by Robin Marantz Henig (Mendel)
History of Genetics: From Prehistoric Times to the redis-covery of Mendel's Laws by Hans Stubbe (MIT press, out of print)	*Lords of the Fly* by Robert E Kohler (*Sociology of Drosophila genetics*) *The Transforming Principle* by Maclyn McCarty
A History of Genetics by Alfred Sturtevant	*Meselson, Stahl, and the Replication of DNA* by Frederic Lawrence Holmes
The Eighth Day of Creation by Horace Freeland Judson (*Focus on molecular biology*)	*We Can Sleep Later:* Alfred Hershey and *The Origins of Molecular Biology* edited by Franlkin W Stahl
The Century of the Gene by Evelyn Fox Keller	*In the Name of Eugenics: Genetics and the Uses of Human Heredity* by Daniel J Kevles
Cracking the Genome: Inside the Race to Unlock Human DNA by Kevin Davies	*The Double Helix* by James Watson
Operators and Promoters	*Rosalind Franklin and DNA* by Anne Sayre
	Rosalind Franklin: The Dark Lady of DNA by Brenda Maddox
	A Feeling for the Organism by Evelyn Fox Keller (Barbara McClintock)
	The Tangled Field: Barbara McClintock's Search for the Patterns of Genetic Control by Nathaniel Comfort (Barbara McClintock)
	Time, Love, Memory by Jonathan Weiner (Seymour Benzer and Drosophila behavioral genetics)

EXERCISE

1. Enumerate the Nobel Prize laureates in the field of genetics.
2. Write briefly about Mendelian laws of inheritance.
3. Who is the father of genetics?
4. Fill in the blanks.
   a. .... and.................. were the 1st to demonstrate the......... in .... of female cat.
   b. .... technology was developed by Fred Sanger.

Introduction

HUMAN GENETICS

The science of heredity has added to the man's precious treasure of inherited characters; physical and mental, both normal as well as abnormal. The expression of these hereditary characters during development as well as life of an individual makes the most fascinating field of study. Thus, in the present era, genetics is one of the new and most significant developing branch of medical science.

There are two main components of this science:

i. *Heredity:* Study of similar traits passed from parents to their offsprings, giving rise to family resemblance.
ii. *Variation:* Study of traits influenced by internal or external forces so that no two individuals are exact replica of each other.

In human beings, the knowledge of genetics can be helpful in many ways:

i. To understand the underlying cause of the disease and means of transmission.
ii. To understand the reasons of normal variations.
iii. To apply the knowledge to the possible means of preventing the genetic disorders through counselling and antenatal diagnosis.
iv. This knowledge can be applied to solve some legal problems like disputed parentage or traits of murderer, etc.

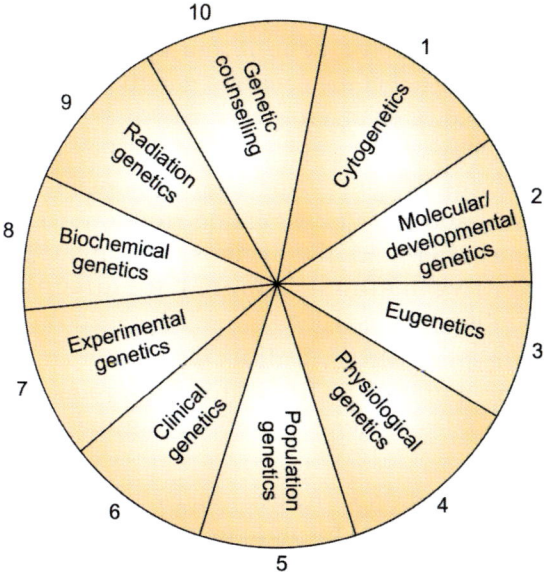

Fig. 2.1: Branches of genetics

BRANCHES OF GENETICS (Fig. 2.1)

1. *Cytogenetics:* The field which gives knowledge of structure of nucleus of a cell and its parts, i.e. chromosomes which normally lie in a condensed form in the nucleus. During cell division, the nuclear membrane disappears and in the metaphase stage the actual number and the detail study of chromosomes is possible. Thus normal chromosomes can be studied and abnormal chromosome and mutation can also be studied in this field.

2. *Molecular/developmental genetics:* The field dealing with the molecular structure of genetic materials and its significance during embryogenesis and functional states of individual during normal as well as developed conditions.

3. *Eugenetics:* The field dealing with the clinical application of principles of heredity for betterment of mankind.

4. *Physiological genetics:* The field elucidates the normal functions of various organelles of a cell governed by the genetic material.

5. *Population genetics:* The field deals with the distribution and behaviour of genetic material in a particular population so that the gene and genotype frequencies are maintained or changed.

6. *Clinical genetics:* The field deals with the application of knowledge of genetic material responsible for certain diseases and their transmission from one generation to another. The field also includes the investigative and preventive methods adopted for diagnosing and preventing the disorders.

7. *Experimental genetics:* It deals with the manipulation of genetic material in living form by recent advanced technologies of genetic engineering and recombinant DNA.

8. *Biochemical genetics:* The field deals with the biochemistry of genetic material for normal metabolic processes. This also includes immunogenetics and blood groups, i.e. genetic material concerned with mechanism of producing antigens and antibodies.

9. *Radiation genetics:* The field deals with the effect of various types of radiation on genetic material producing various diseases.

10. *Genetic counselling:* The branch deals with the immediate and practical preventive and social health promotional measures in problems of genetic disorders. The counsellor named as *medical geneticist* can deal with matters pertaining to the causation, incidence, risks of recurrence of inherited defects, radiation hazards, mutant viral strains in biological warfare, some newer drugs including the anticancer drugs which can cure genetic problems due to mutation, also come under the purview of counsellor are also seen in human beings.

EXERCISE

1. Write briefly about the components of human genetics.
2. In what ways the study of genetics helps human beings?
3. Write a short note on genetic counselling.

4. Fill in the blanks.
   a. Study of .... and .... chromosomes is called cytogenetics.
   b. .... of mankind with .... application is ....eugenetics.
   c. .... and .... of genetic.................. in a particular population is called..................
   d. .... structure of genetic.................. during.................. is called as molecular and developmental genetics.

5. Match the following.

i. Immunogenetics	a. Experimental genetics
ii. Transmission	b. Physiological genetics
iii. Genetic disorder	c. Medical geneticist
iv. Organelles of cell	d. Biochemical genetics
v. Recombination DNA	e. Clinical genetics

3

Cytogenetics

NORMAL CHROMOSOMES

Genes, the units of inheritance, are located on the chromosomes of the gametes. They are passed from parents to progeny through successive generations after fertilization. The term chromosome was introduced into the scientific library by Waldeyer in 1888.

The number of chromosomes is fixed in each cell and varies from species to species. In human beings, the total number is 46 or 23 pairs given the name as diploid ($2n$), as the number in the gametes of both male as well as female is just the half of it, i.e. 23 and is thus called as haploid (n). It is only after fertilization that the diploid number is maintained. Twenty two of the chromosomes in haploid set are named as autosomes (Fig. 3.1) and each has its homologous or matching chromosome in other gamete. The remaining one pair of chromosome in each gamete is called as sex chromosome (Fig. 3.2) which are not exactly matching and in females it is called X-chromosome while in males it is called Y-chromosome. Therefore, the female cells will have XX while the male cells will have XY chromosomes which are not exactly matching as far as the morphology and structure are concerned.

Human chromosomes are rod shaped, V-shaped or J-shaped or twisted in various spiral or curved shape visible only during cell divison. They vary in their length from 4–6 μ and are shortest during metaphase stage of cell division. Chemically each chromosome is essentially a DNA protein package, capable of self replication and retains its structural and functional integrity through all successive division of any cell type.

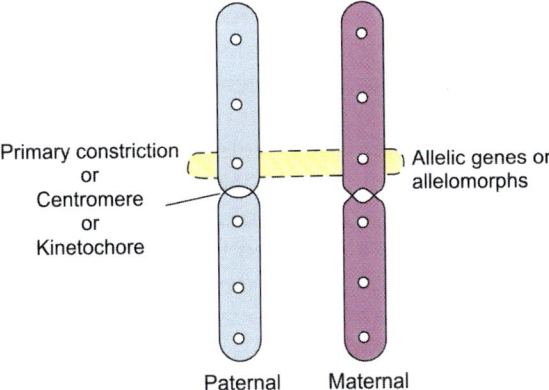

Fig. 3.1: A pair of homologous chromosomes

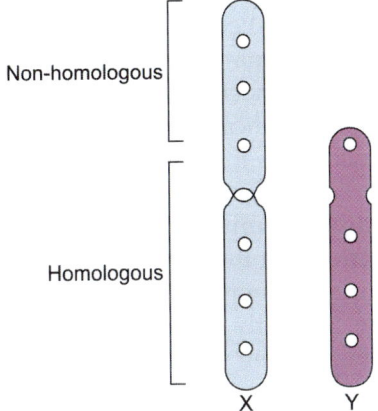

Fig. 3.2: Sex chromosome in male

Chemical constituents are:

1. DNA
2. RNA
3. Histone
4. Acidic proteins

STRUCTURE (GROSS)

Each pair of homologous chromosomes show a common basic structure. One chromosome is made up of two identical parallel filaments called chromatids, which are held together at a narrow constricted region, usually pale staining, known as primary constriction, or centromere or kinetochore (Fig. 3.1). This structure is visible only during metaphase stage of cell division. Each chromosome gets attached to spindle by kinetochore during cell division. Secondary constrictions are also found along the length of some of the chromosomes. These constrictions can be distinguished from primary constrictions by the absence of marked angular deviation of the chromosomal segment which is named as *terminal satellite body*. Such chromosomes are named as SAT chromosomes (Fig. 3.3) and the satellites and the filaments of secondary constriction are constant in shape and size in a particular chromosome. These constrictions are said to be responsible for the formation of nucleoli during condensed stage of nucleus and thus these chromosomes are also called as nucleolar organizers. Most of the chromosomes in human beings vary in their length from 4–6 μ, and they are the shortest during metaphase stage of cell division. Functional significance of chromosomes lie in carrying the instructions necessary for proper organisation and working of various tissues and thus organs of body. Each cell in its complete set of diploid number of chromosomes carries all the inherited instructions on their threads or filaments known as chromonemata or genonemata and the set of instruction is called as genome. Secondly, the chromosomes also control the cell activity during protein synthesis.

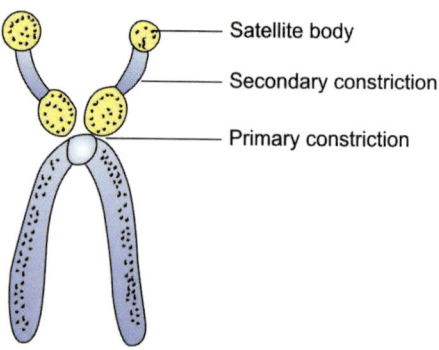

Satellite body

Secondary constriction

Primary constriction

Fig. 3.3: A pair of SAT chromosome

CLASSIFICATION (GROSS)—GENERAL

All the chromosomes can be classified as given below.

i. Based on the *number of the centromeres*:
  a. *Acentric:* When there is absence of centromere, not seen in human beings.
  b. *Monocentric:* Only one centromere, found in human beings.
  c. *Dicentric:* Two centromeres, one in each chromatid, seen only during chromosomal anomalies.
  d. *Polycentric:* More than two centromeres.

ii. Based on the *position of the centromere,* i.e. the location of the centromere (Fig. 3.4)
  a. *Telocentric:* When the centromere is situated at one end of chromosomes so that each chromatid has only one arm. These are not found in human beings.
  b. *Acrocentric:* When the centromere is situated near one end of chromosome being subterminal in position, so that one arm is longer than the other in each chromatid. The short arm in some of these possess satellite bodies.
  c. *Sub-metacentric:* When the centromere is situated slightly away from the mid-point of chromosome, i.e. in between the midpoint and end of each chromatid again giving rise to two unequal arms.

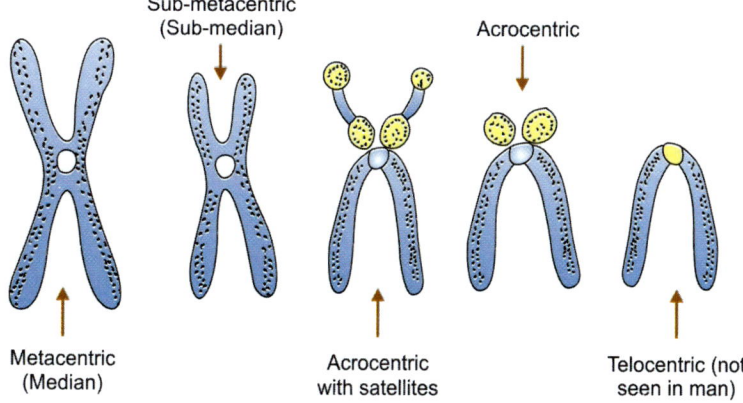

Fig. 3.4: Types of chromosomes (according to the position of centromere)

d. *Metacentric:* When the centromere is located in the centre, so that the two arms of each chromatid are almost equal in size.

CLASSIFICATION—SPECIFIC

Human chromosomes have been classified for their individual identification by the total length, the position of centromere, banding pattern, by the presence of satellite bodies and other morphological features. By the Denver–London system, all the autosomal chromosomes have been numbered from 1 to 22 in decreasing order of length or size and the sex chromosomes being put to distinct label as X and Y. There is another modified classification by Denver, when all the chromosomes including sex chromosomes are put in a total of seven groups from A-G in order of their decreasing length but position of centromere in each group being same. The chromosomes arranged in such a manner are called to form a karyotype. Some morphological features for identification of individual chromosomes must be kept in mind while preparing a karyotype like all the longest metacentric chromosomes are grouped in A group while group G contains shortest acrocentric chromosomes. The seven groups are as follows (Fig. 3.5).

Group A	Contains automsomes number 1, 2 and 3—large metacentric (number 2 is more towards sub-metacentric)
Group B	Contains autosomes number 4 and 5—large sub-metacentric.
Group C	Contains autosomes number 6 to 12 and X-chromosome—medium sized sub-metacentric (No. 6, 7, 8 and 11 are more towards metacentric).
Group D	Contains autosomes number 13 to 15—medium acrocentric with satellite bodies on short arms.
Group E	Contains autosomes number 16 to 18—small sub-metacentric.
Group F	Contains autosomes number 19 and 20—small metacentric.

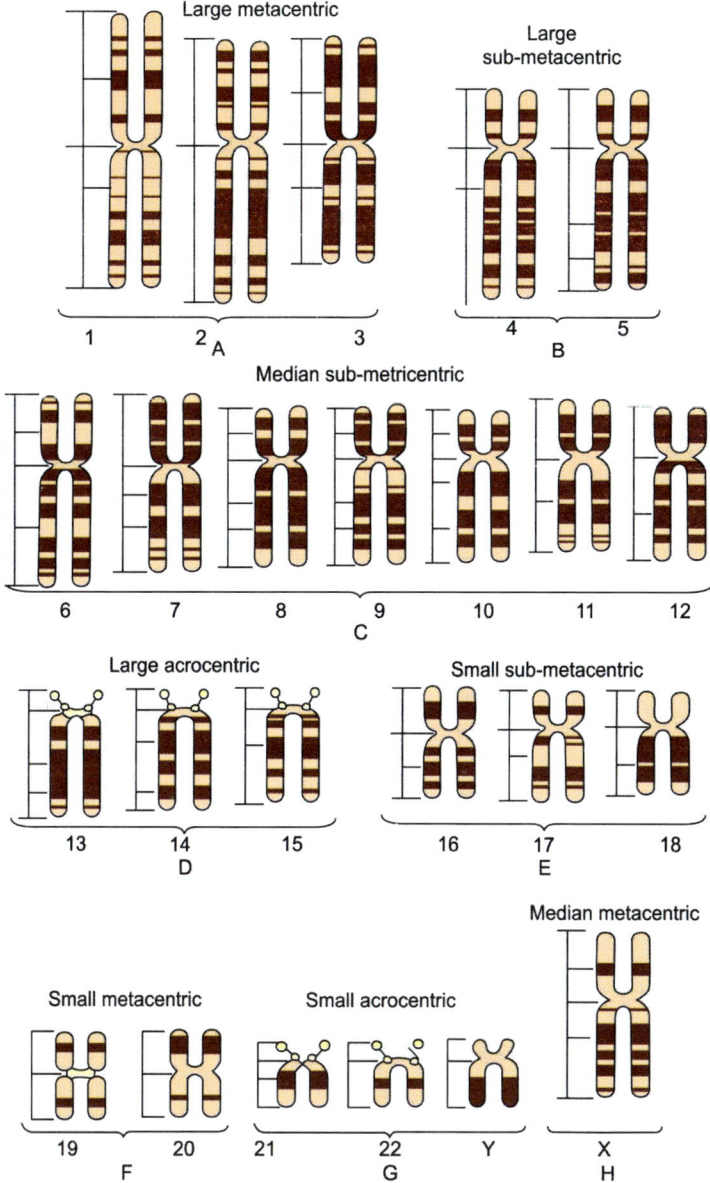

Fig. 3.5: Banding pattern of individual chromosomes set for whole haploid autosomes and pair of sex chromosomes shown in groups C and G

Group G   Contains autosomes number 21 and 22 and Y-chromosome—small acrocentric with satellite bodies on 21 and 22 only and not on Y-chromosome.

A more accurate method of identifying each individual chromosome was introduced in 1971 and later in 1975 in Paris known as Paris nomenclature. The chromosomes can be individually identified by their banding pattern. The bands have been numbered on the short arm and long arm of each chromsome named as p and q respectively (even in metacentric chromosomes also both the arms are not exactly equal). Both the arms are first divided into various regions numbered 1, 2, etc. starting from centromere and each region is further subdivided into numbered band (Table 3.1). For example, 1-q, 2, 1 means band number 1 in the second region of the long arm of chromosomes number 1 (Fig. 3.6).

Bands serving as landmarks which divide the chromosomes into cytologically defined regions.

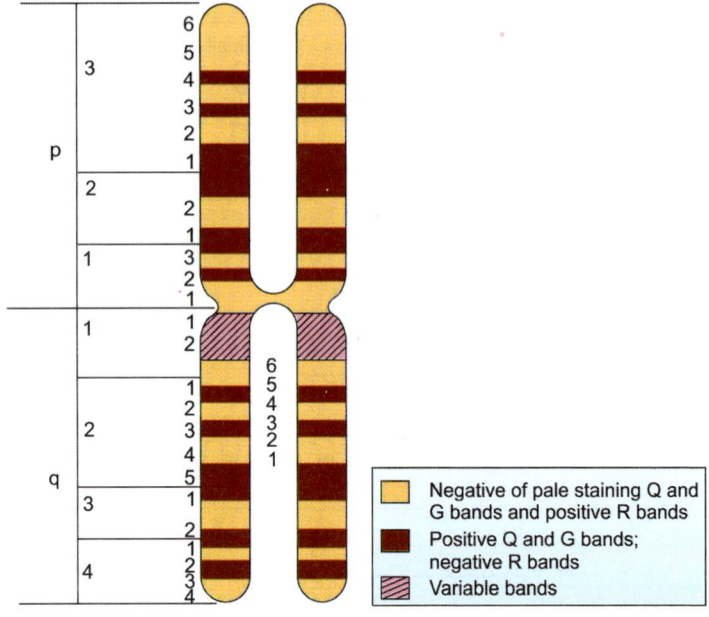

Fig. 3.6: Q, G and R bands in chromosome number 1

METHODS OF STUDYING THE CHROMOSOMES

1. *Techniques which are used to study the complete chromosome complement of an individual:* For complete chromosomal analysis (Fig. 3.7), cells which divide rapidly in culture medium are used. The most commonly used cells are fibroblasts of skin, bone marrow cells and peripheral blood lymphocytes and even exfoliated amniotic fluid cells from a pregnant woman. Viable cells can also be obtained within a few hours of death of individual or following an abortion.

From peripheral blood, the lymphocytes are separated and added to a culture medium with phytohaemagglutinin added to it. This stimulates the leucocytes to divide. The cells are cultured under aseptic measures at 37 °C for about three days. The cell division is arrested by adding a small amount of colchicine to the culture. After one hour of adding colchicine, a

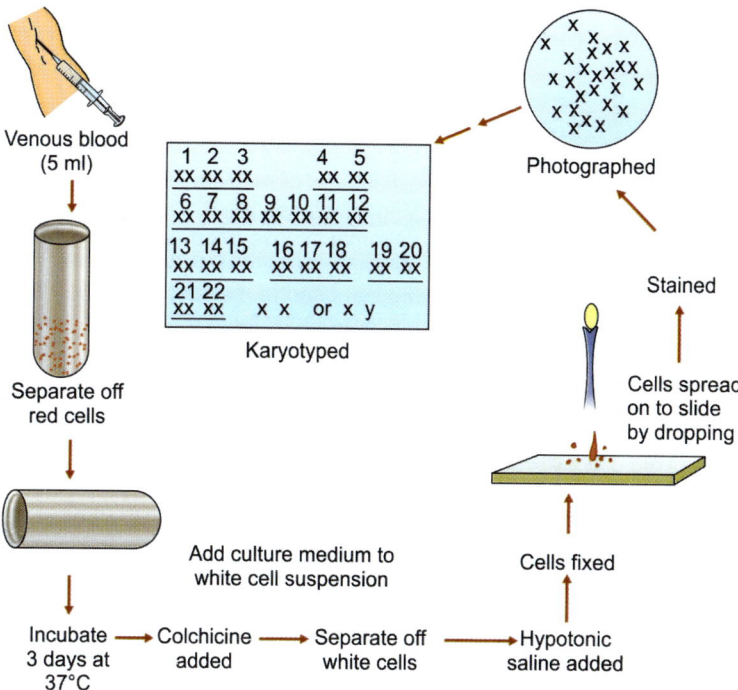

Fig. 3.7: The preparation of a karyotype

Table 3.1: Chromosome* bands

Chromosome no.	Arm	Number of region	Landmarks**
1	p	3	Proximal band of medium intensity (2,1), median band of medium intensity (3,1)
	q	4	Proximal negative band (2,1) distal to variable region, median intense band (3,1)/ distal medium band (4,1)
2	p	2	Median negative band (2,1)
	q	3	Proximal negative band (2,1)/distal negative band (3,1)
3	p	2	Median negative band (2,1)
	q	2	Median negative band (2,1)
4	q	3	Proximal negative band (2, 1)/ distal negative band (3,1)
5	q	3	Median band of medium intensity (2,1), distal negative band (3,1)
6	p	2	Median negative band (2,1)
	q	2	Median negative band (2,1)
7	p	2	Distal medium band (2,1)
	q	3	Proximal medium band (2, 1)/ median band of medium intensity (3,1)
8	p	2	Median negative band (2,1)
	q	2	Median intense band (2,1)
9	q	3	Median band of medium intensity (2, 1)/ distal band of medium intensity (3,1)
	p	2	Median intense band
10	q	2	Proximal intense band (2,1)
11	q	2	Median negative band (2,1)
12	q	2	Median band of medium intensity (2,1)
13	q	3	Median intense band (2, 1), distal intense band (3,1)
14	q	3	Proximal intense band (2, 1), distal medium band (3,1)
15	q	2	Median intense band (2,1)
16	q	2	Median band of medium intensity (2,1)
17	q	2	Proximal negative band (2,1)
18	q	2	Median negative band (2,1)
21	q	2	Median intense band (2,1)
X	p	2	Proximal medium band (2,1)
	q	2	Proximal medium band (2,1)

*The omission of an entire chromosome or chromosome arm indicates that either both arms or the arm in question consists of only one region, delimited by the centromere and the end of the chromosome arm.

**The numbers in parentheses are the regions and band numbers.

hypotonic solution is added to swell the cells and allow the chromosomes to spread on the slide and stained with Giemsa stain. Now a high powered photomicrograph is taken and each chromosome is cut out from photograph, arranged in pairs in decreasing order of size and numbered 1–22 and two sex chromosomes indicated separately, forming a karyotype. The whole process is called karyotyping. The karyotyping will tell only the number and gross features of chromosomes but it is difficult to detect the structural abnormalities of chromosomes, however, minor it may be. The latest methods of study are by chromosomal banding by general and special techniques for full range or restricted range of bands respectively throughout the chromosomal complement.

T Casperson was the scientist to discover the stain *quinacrine mustard*—a fluorescent DNA-binding compound for chromosome banding. When the karyotyping is being done after making the slide the cells are stained by Giemsa stain, or quinacrine hydrochloride or mustard or the slide is treated with trypsin prior to Giemsa stain to denature the chromosomal protein for general or special banding pattern. According to the stain used and the method used for banding, following names have been assigned:

i. *Giemsa banding* or *G-banding* which shows similar banding pattern during mitosis and meiosis. The bands are seen as dark and light areas when the slides are pretreated with trypsin prior to Giemsa staining.

ii. *Quinacrine banding* or *Q-banding:* The slides are stained with quinacrine hydrochloride or quinacrine mustard and when examined by fluorescent microscope each pair of chromosome shows specific bright and dim bands, the bright bands corresponding to the dark bands of G-banding. Here also there is identical pattern seen during mitosis and meiosis.

iii. *Reverse banding:* R-banding, when pretreatment with heat is given prior to Giemsa staining and thus the resulting dark and light bands are the reverse of those produced by G-banding. Here also there is identical pattern seen during mitosis and meiosis.

iv. *Special banding methods:* C-banding is done by extraction of DNA by alkali from the chromosome. Highly repetitive DNA sequences resist such extraction.

These resistant sequences are usually found adjacent to the centromere of all chromosomes and distal portion of Y-chromosome. These bands represent thus highly repetitive, non-transcribed DNA known in nuclei heterochromatin.

C-banding can also be brought about by staining with the A-T specific DNA ligand, Hoechst 33258, producing intense fluorescence of highly A-T rich satellite DNA's found in the C-band regions.

v. *Cd-banding:* When a protein associated with centromere is stained and site of Cd band is seen in every chromosome, i.e. centromere.

vi. *G11 banding:* It is done by using Giemsa stain very highly alkaline pH, i.e. 11 or even higher. This brings about only eosin component of Giemsa stain to be effective producing red staining of proteins on the short arms of acrocentric chromosomes.

vii. *AgN banding silver staining of RNA:* The bands represent the nucleolus organizing regions, present on almost all the ten chromosomes of D and G group (No. 13, 14, 15, 21 and 22) with a range of three to all the ten chromosomes. These bands mark the sites of transcriptionally active ribosomal RNA genes.

In males, group G includes Y chromosome which differs from the other chromosomes of same group in three features:

a. It is usually the longest in group G.

b. The long arms are usually parallel to each other being divergent in the other members of the group.

c. There are no satellite bodies in short arms.

The X-chromosome is of group C and can be distinguished from other members of the group by special banding techniques. In a karyotype, each chromosome can be identified by using certain parameters which are:

i. Shape of the chromosome.

ii. Length of the chromosome.

iii. Centromeric index: Which is expressed as the ratio of the short arm length to the total chromsomes length, i.e. centromeric index—short arm length: Total chromosome length.

In a metacentric chromosome, the index is 0.5.

iv. Proportion of the arms: It is the ratio between the long and short arms of the chromosome. In a typical metacentric chromosome, this ratio is 1:1.

2. *Methods to obtain information about sex chromosomes constitution only.* The second technique to give information regarding the sex chromosome can be applied for:

i. Study of sex chromatin or Barr body.

ii. Study of flourescent bodies in buccal smear.

iii. Study of drumsticks in polymorphonuclear leucocytes.

In 1949, Barr and Bertman were the first to describe a body usually lying near the nucleolus of nuclei of neurones of cat. It was named as sex chromatin or Barr body; it was found to be present in females only with the frequency of about 85% in nervous tissue, in whole mounts of amniotic or chorionic epithelium it may be as high as 96%, and in oral smears the frequency varies between 20 to 50% in normal females.

Sex chromatin represents one of the two X-chromosomes of cells of females which is genetically inactive. It shows condensed chromatin during the resting phase of cell cycle. It is seen under the microscope as a small chromocentre heavily stained with basic dyes in the interphase nucleus. It can be found attached to the nucleolus as in nerve cell (Fig. 3.8a) attached to nuclear membrane as in cells of epidermis of buccal mucosa (Fig. 3.8b) and seen as a nuclear expansion in about 3% of neutrophil leucocytes forming a small rod called as drumstick (Fig. 3.8c).

The sex chromatin appears during the second week of development of female embryo; MF Lyon formulated a hypothesis stating that in the female cells, one of the X-chromosome is inactivated during the early development periods and only one of the two X-chromosomes is actually genetically active. The inactive X can be either paternal or

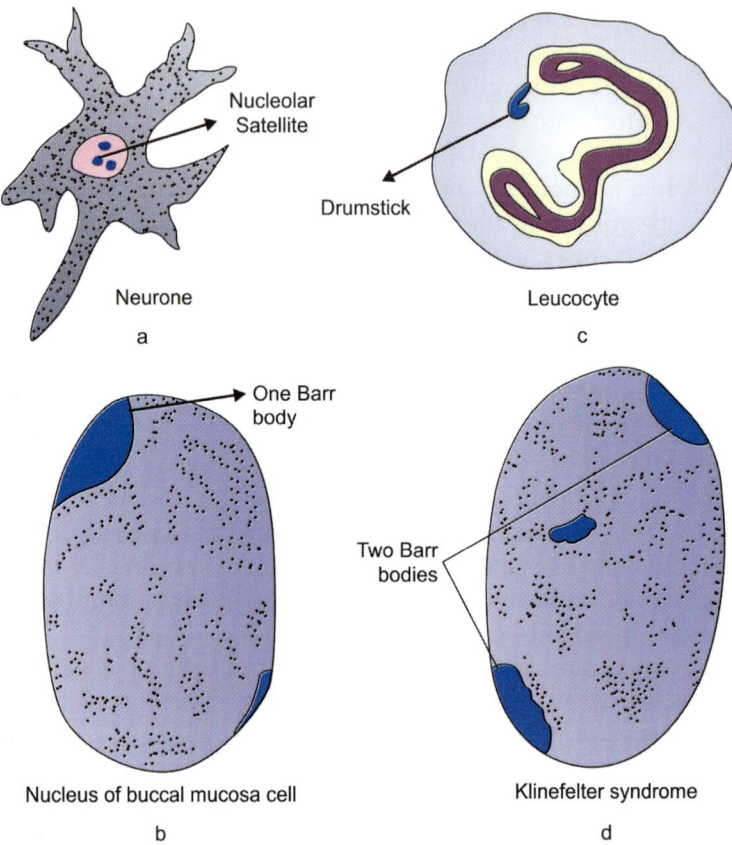

Fig. 3.8: Sex chromatin in various cells

maternal in different cells of same individual. Thus it occurs at random during embryonic period but fixed for a particular cell line. The observation made by Lyon are:

i. The female cells have the Barr body while the male cells do not have it.

ii. The number of Barr bodies is one less than the total number of X-chromosomes. Thus a normal female has only one Barr body while Klinefelter's syndrome (XXXY) has 2 Barr bodies, and so on (Fig. 3.8d).

iii. Sex linked for practical purposes are X-linked genes. In males as there is only one X-chromosome and the traits present on X-chromosome will appear uniformly phenotypically depending on the genotype. In females if the genes are homozygous in both X-chromosomes the traits will appear uniformly being paternal or maternal in origin. However, some interesting findings are noticed in females having heterozygous genotype. Instead of expression of the traits uniformly, there is a mixture of expressed traits, accounting for the phenomenon of random lyonization rendering an X-chromosome— paternal or maternal, inactive in all the cells of body differently. Thus X-linked recessive inheritance will be expressed commonly in males and an X-linked dominant trait, rarer, both males and females will express the trait equally.

Evidence to Explain Lyon's Hypothesis .

i. Some known enzymes like glucose-6-phosphate dehydrogenase or antihaemophilic globulin, produced by genes located on the X-chromosomes are equal in two sexes. Inactivation of one of the two chromosomes does not produce any change in the production of these enzymes.

ii. Females possessing an abnormal X-linked gene present only on one X-chromsomes (heterozygous) and do express abnormalities when there is total lyonization as this abnormal gene is functional in most of the cells.

iii. When the cells of women are cultured specially in tissue culture, two different clonal populations can be seen—one with active X and another with the alternative inactive X.

There are some facts that do no confirm to Lyon's hypothesis, e.g. abnormal phenotype of XO and XXY individuals who physically differ from normal XX females or XY males, respectively. Whereas, by reasoning out practically XO females should be normal, since there is one X in females which is active and thus effectively XO, and similarly XXY males should be normal being XY effectively. The possible explanation is that the sexual differentiation occurs at early embryonic period before the inactivation of the X-chromosome. Thus XO, XX,

XXY and XY are not equal as far as their developmental control is concerned. Another possibility is that the inactivation does not involve the whole of the chromosome but only part of it, and the nonactivated part carries the genes that determine the phenotypic difference between XO and XX.

BEHAVIOUR OF CHROMOSOME DURING CELL DIVISION

All the cells in the body multiply by division involving both nucleus and cytoplasm. The division of cell for multiplication is essential for:

i. Embryogenesis.
ii. Postnatal growth and replacement of dead cells.

The cell division involves two well defined steps:

i. Karyokinesis–division of nucleus, i.e. chromosomal division.
ii. Cytokinesis–division of cytoplasm, i.e. normally the cytoplasmic constituents are distributed equally in the two daughter cells.

The cells are required to divide, influenced by certain factors deciding the rate and time of division. The factors like rate, demand, time along with hazardous effects of radiations and chemical substances will always influence the cell divisions. There will be rapid cell division of epithelial tissue for replacement as compared to nervous tissue where the neurones once formed are never replaced. The rate of cell division is also dependent on the demand of body for a tissue, e.g. it is maximum during healing of a wound and it has to be in a co-ordinated way. The defects in this co-ordination of demand for growth and replacement can lead to lesser growth or over growth. Some hormones also influence the cell division leading to diurnal variation, e.g. epidermal cells of skin usually divide at night because during day time the epinephrine in blood forms a complex with epidermal chalone which inhibits cell division. This has been named as diurnal mitotic rhythm. Similarly, cell division is inhibited by exposure to radiations affecting the regeneration and failure of chromatids to separate. Chemical agents like colchicine and viblastin, etc. prevent the formation of a spindle microtubules and thus arresting the cell division at a particular time. This property has been utilized significantly in cytogenetic study during metaphase of cell division. The exact control mechanism of cell division is ill defined. However, following observations may be of some use for better understanding:

a. Local control—during early embryonic period there is exchange of metabolites amongst different cell groups by simple diffusion to either stimulate or depress the cell division.

b. Hormonal control—during later period of development certain hormones take over the role of local factors e.g. thyroid hormone and corticosteroid affect the metabolic rate and protein synthesis respectively.

c. A chemical substance called chalone has been found to be existing in normal cells. It is protein in nature with molecular weight of 30,000 to 50,000 daltons. It is thought to be inhibitory for cell division. This chemical is believed to be cell specific but not species specific. In wound healing, because of the cell damage the concentration of chalones falls leading to stimulation of cell division but as soon as the normal level of chalones is restored the cell division is again inhibited.

THE CELL CYCLE

All the cells of body show a definite pattern for multiplication, so that the final stage of division ends at the beginning of the first stage, repeating the whole sequence again and again. This is called cell cycle (Fig. 3.9). Depending on the demand, the cell division called as mitosis may repeat without any resting period but usually there is a phase of longer or shorter duration called as interphase. Most of the body cells are seen in interphase of cell cycle. It is during the interphase that the cell prepares itself for next division. There are usually three stages during interphase after the mitosis (M phase lasting for 1–3 hour).

1. *First gap phase (G-1):* It is also called as pre-duplication phase. It is during this phase, most cells of body exist and function (Time: 8–11 hours).

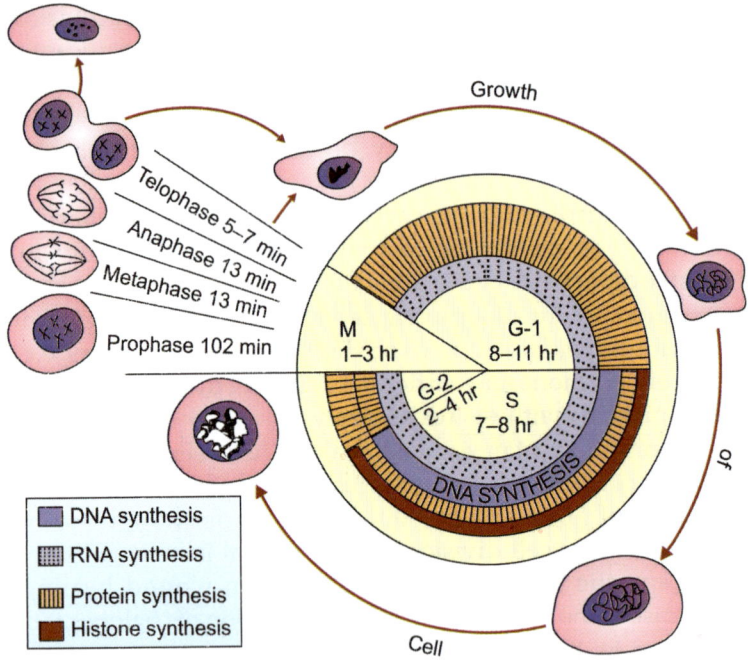

Fig. 3.9: The cell cycle

2. *DNA duplication phase (S-phase)*—Synthesis of DNA occurs during this phase and lasts for usually 7–8 hours.
3. *Second gap phase (G-2)*—Post-duplication phase lasting for only half an hour to 2–4 hours.

The time taken by a cell to divide is called as generation time and the total duration as well as the duration of various phases in a cycle varies in the animal kingdom from tissues to tissues.

The karyokinesis part of the cell division is of two types:

a. *Direct:* When the nucleus is constricted in the middle and then divides into two, so that the nuclear material is distributed at random in the resultant cells. This type of cell division occurs only during some pathological conditions.
b. *Indirect:* When the nuclear material, i.e. chromosomes show some characteristics changes in a definite pattern. This is further subdivided into mitosis or homotypical division, where the nuclear material first doubles itself and then is

distributed equally in each of the daugther cell; thus having same amount of nuclear material, meiosis or heterotypical division, where the nuclear material is exactly halved in such a manner that daughter cell has similar nuclear material but half of the amount.

In higher animals the indirect division occurs, in somatic cells it is mitosis, while in sex cells it is meiosis (Table 3.2).

Table 3.2: Differences between meiosis and mitosis	
Meiosis	*Mitosis*
1. It always occurs in germimal cells only during gametogenesis.	1. It occurs in all the cells of body somatic as well as germinal but during maturation of latter, it does not occur.
2. The whole division is completed by two sequences resulting in two daughter cells from one germinal cell.	2. The division is completed by one sequence and results in two daughter cells.
3. Daughter cells are not same as the parent cell because of crossing over and exchange of genetic material and reduction in number chromosomes to half, i.e. haploid.	3. Daughter cells resemble the parent cells because of no exchange of genetic material and number of chromosomes is also same, i.e. diploid.
4. The various phases, prophase metaphase, anaphases and telophase occur twice with varying duration resulting in four daughter cells.	4. The phases occur only once to produce two daughter cells.
5. Cytokinesis is not necessary to occur in telophase I but normally extends to second meiotic division.	5. Cytokinesis always occur after each division.
6. Synthesis of DNA occurs during S-phase of interphase of first meiotic division and no synthesis occurs during short interphase of second meiotic division.	6. Synthesis of DNA during S-phase of interphase

MITOSIS

During mitosis (Fig. 3.10), the exact replica of the parent cell is produced having the same genomenata in the daughter cells (lasting for 1–3 hours). In the actively dividing cell, the new DNA is synthesized during S-phase of interphase so that the DNA amount is doubled with the number of chromosomes still diploid. This DNA amount is equally distributed in the two daughter cells during mitosis so that the DNA amount as well as the number of chromosomes is diploid in both the cells. Mitosis consists of the following four stages.

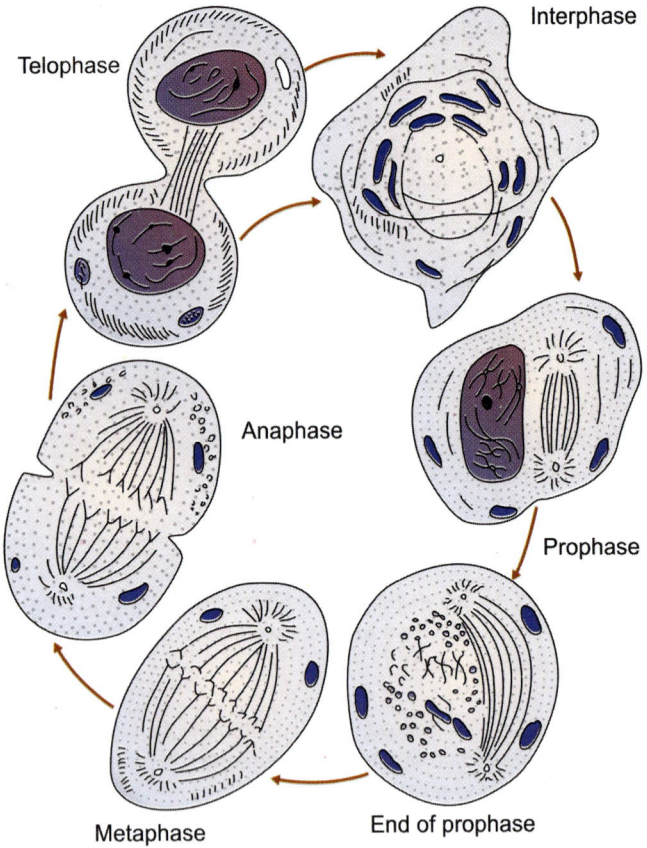

Fig. 3.10: Stages of cell division in mitosis

1. *Prophase:* Lasting for about 102 minutes, consists of following features:
   i. The chromatin material of nucleus gets shortened or condensed so that chromosomes can be recognized, each made up of two chromatids joined at centromere.
   ii. The centrioles in the cytoplasm move away from each other to be placed at two poles of cell.
   iii. Microtubules are synthesized between two centrioles forming a spindle and radiate to form astral rays.
   iv. The nucleoli disappear.
   v. The nuclear membrane disappears.

2. *Metaphase:* Chromosomes are shortened and condensed and thus best visualized. The time taken is about 13 minutes.
   i. The microtubules synthesized during prophase forming a spindle moves towards the centre of cell.
   ii. The chromosomes move to the equator of spindle.
   iii. The chromosomes are attached to spindle at the centromere on the equator, limbs of chromosomes not lying in the plane of equator.
   iv. When seen from both the poles of cell the chromosomes appear as a star, like ring.
   v. The other organnelles, like mitochondria, are distributed equally in the margins of cell.

3. *Anaphase* (again, upward, backward): Time is about 9 minutes (shortest phase).
   i. There is splitting of the double metaphasic centromere so that each chromatid from a split original chromosome moves to opposite side.
   ii. All the chromosomes are grouped at each pole of cell and in both groups the number of chromosome is diploid.
   iii. The initiation of cytoplasmic division is seen as infolding of cell membrane at equator.
      The longitudinal splitting, by the formation of cleavage furrow in each chromosome is brought about by shortening of the microtubules and the repelling force of split chromatids.

4. *Telophase:* It represents the last stage of mitosis when the following events occur. Time is 57 minutes.

  i. The visible coiled chromosome becomes uncoiled or lengthens or are extended.

  ii. The nuclear membrane reappears.

  iii. The nucleoli reappear.

  iv. The cytoplasmic cleavage at the equator deepens and ultimately divides the cell into two.

  v. The spindle remnants also disintegrate and disappear.

A cell seen in any phase of mitosis during routine examination of tissues or organs are said to be mitotic figures. These figures are usually seen in places where growth is occurring, or maintenance of cell population is essential, e.g. bone marrow, lining membrane of intestine, or sites where repair process is in progress, e.g. fracture of bones, and finally at places of abnormal growth, e.g. cancer.

The abnormal mitosis, when the two chromatids move towards one pole, results in lagging of chromosomes leading to a condition called non-dysjunction. Radiation increases the chances of such events due to damage of chromosomes and even mitosis may be completely inhibited. Chemical substances like colchicine and its derivatives also inhibit mitosis by inhibiting the microtubule spindle formation during metaphase. The advantage of this knowledge has been of great help in chromosomal studies.

MEIOSIS

Meiosis (Fig. 3.11) takes place in gonads during gametogenesis only. It consists of two successive divisions called first meiotic and second meiotic divisions. It is during the interphase of first meiotic division that the DNA is replicated in the usual manner leading to tetraploid amount of DNA in diploid number of chromosomes, and during first meiotic division only the amount of DNA is reduced to diploid amount in each chromosome and chromosome number is also halved to haploid. In meiosis II, the DNA in each new daughter cell is reduced to haploid, the chromosome number remaining haploid.

The chief stages in the meiotic cycle

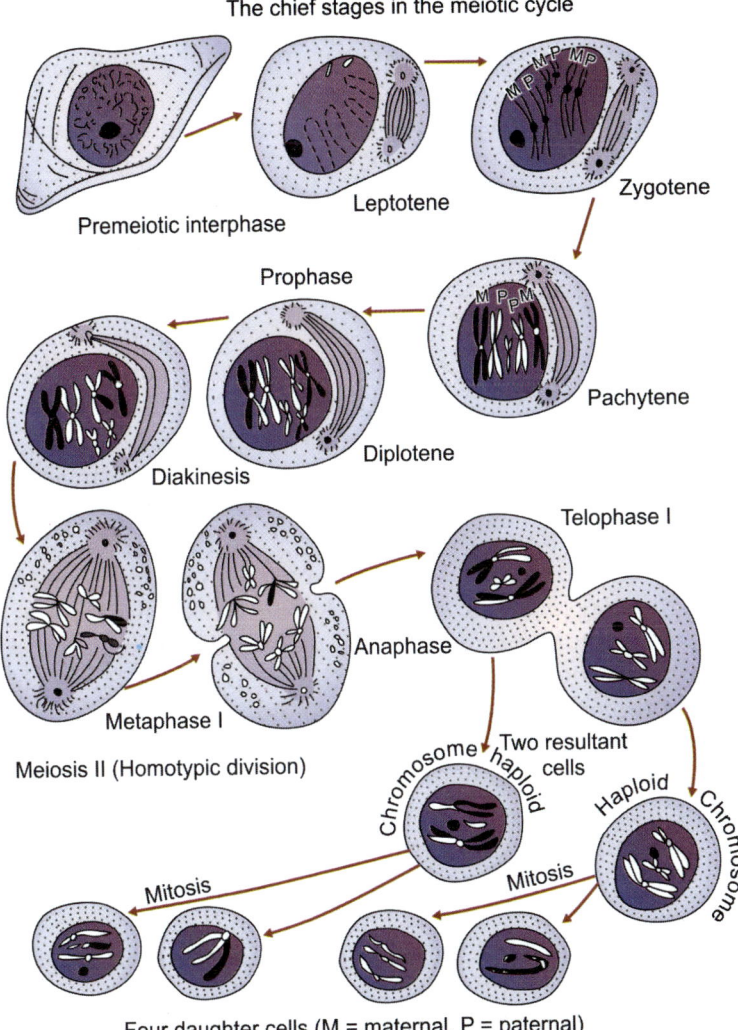

Fig. 3.11: Stages of cell division in meiosis

Both first and second meiotic divisions can be further sub-divided into the same four stages—prophase, metaphase, anaphase and telophase—each with few differences in the behaviour of chromosomes and duration of phase.

Meiosis I

1. *Interphase:* The DNA content of chromosome is doubled, i.e. it is tetraploid.

2. *Prophase:* This phase is of longer duration and complex and differs distinctly from meiotic prophase. It can be divided into following five stages:

   i. *Leptotene stage:* The thin chromosomal threads shorten and become thick so that they are visible as individual threads. One end of each thread is attached to the nuclear membrane. Each thread shows a beaded appearance throughout their length known as chromomeres. The separate chromatoids can not be seen.

   ii. *Zygotene stage:* The two members of a homologous pair of chromosome come to lie side by side forming a bivalent. This pairing is point to point so that the same regions of the chromosome lie in contact. The process is called synapsis or conjugation. In the case of males, the X and Y pair only in limited segments known as pairing segments, the remaining regions are differential segments. A synaptinemal complex in the form of fibrillar band occupying a space of about 100 nm is found by electron microscope to hold the two homologous chromosomes together.

   iii. *Pachytene stage:* More shortening and thickening of the chromosomes occurs so that now the two chromatids joining at centromere is clearly visible. Thus each pair of chromosome consists of four chromatids called as tetrad. An important event now takes place, i.e. two chromatids one from each bivalent becomes coiled around each other thereby crossing at several levels—the phenomenon is known as crossing over or recombination or chiasma, where exchange of genetic material between the two homologous chromosomes take place, leading to a large variety of the final genetic make up of an individual. Precise timing and nature of DNA exchange is uncertain and it can occur as early as during the S phase of the previous interphase.

iv. *Diplotene stage:* Now the homologous chromosomes move away to separate except at chiasmata points. Later the chiasmata breaks. Normally, atleast one chiasmata is formed between each pair but upto even five have been observed. Sometimes the chiasmata move towards the end of chromatids.

In human meiosis, primary oocytes become diplotene by the fifth month of intrauterine life and remain in this stage till prior to ovulation.

v. *Diakinesis stage:* The remaining chiasma finally break separating the two chromatids, but still bivalent. The bivalents now move away from each other and spread against the nuclear membrane.

The nucleoli disappears. Spindle and asteral rays form as in mitosis. The end of prophase is characterized by the disappearance of nuclear membrane and bivalent chromosomes moving towards the equatorial plane of cell.

Metaphase-I: It is similar to metaphase of mitosis, the difference being only that it is the homologous pair of chromosomes which lie parallel on the equator of the spindle of microtubules with one member on either side of equator, i.e. it is the bivalent tetrad chromosome.

Anaphase-I: It differs from anaphase of mitosis in that the centromere does not split. So that one whole chromosome of homologous pair move apart to reach the opposite poles of cell. This results in haploid number of chromosomes in each daughter cell, i.e. 23 chromosomes consisting of two chromatids.

Telophase-I: As there is random positioning of maternal and paternal bivalent chromosomes, there is random assortment of maternal and paternal chromosomes in each daughter cells produced by cytoplasmic division during telophase.

Meiosis II

There is a brief interval in the form of unique interphase during which there is no DNA synthesis. Otherwise there is no difference from mitosis, except that the two separating chromatids during anaphase are genetically dissimilar. This is because of formation during the first meiotic division.

Significance of Meiosis

  i. Meiosis or reduction division is essential during gametogenesis.

 ii. The chromosomal number characteristic for human beings will be retained after fertilization only.

iii. The exchange of genetic material leads to formation of new combinations and thus new traits.

The essentiality of reduction division can be explained as under.

- If the number of chromosomes remain same during gametogenesis then each gamete will have diploid (2*n*), i.e.

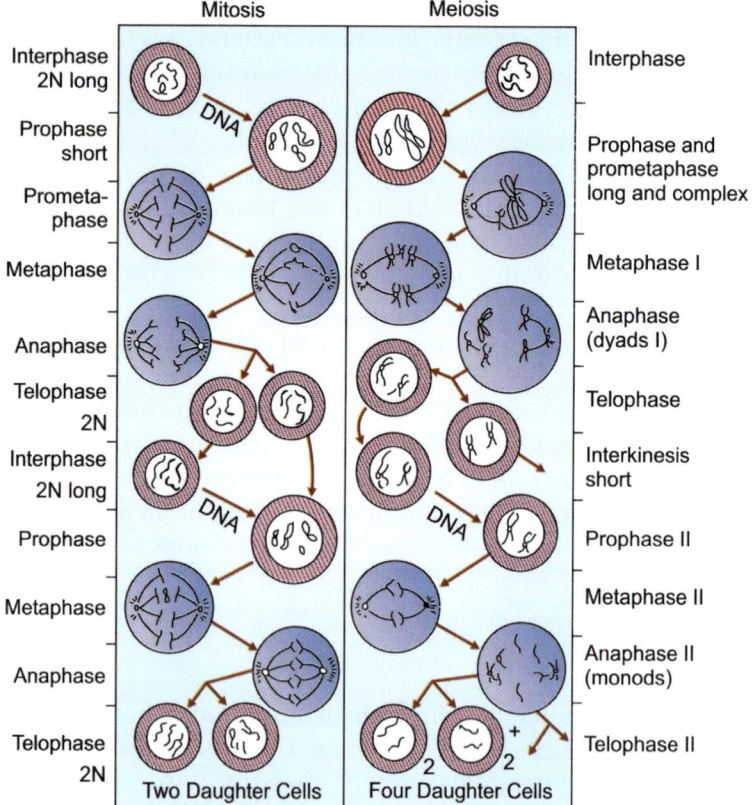

Fig. 3.12: Differences between mitosis and meiosis (schematic)

46 chromosomes and the resultant zygote will have tetraploid (4*n*), i.e. 92 chromosomes.

- This is non-specific for human beings and thus a different creature, if at all, will be formed.
- The repetition of the same cell division resulting in multiples of chromosome number for future generations can give rise to a new species every time, which is significant during evolutionary history (Fig. 3.12).

EXERCISE

1. Write short notes on:
   a. Sex chromosomes
   b. Primary constrictions
   c. Nucleolar organisers
   d. Autosomes
2. Classify chromosomes based on:
   a. Position of centromere
   b. Morphology
3. Write in tabulated form, the differences between mitosis and meiosis.
4. Fill in the blanks.
   a. .... of cell division is of two types .... and .... the later is further of two types .... and ....
   b. The resting period during .... cycle is known as ....
   c. Most cells of body function during .... phase of cell cycle, lasting for .... hours.
   d. DNA .... occurs during.................. phase of cell cycle, lasting for .... hours.
5. Enumerate the basic components of structure of a chromosome.
6. Draw a diagram to show the stages for making a karyotype.
7. Enumerate the various banding methods used for individual chromosomal structure.
8. Match the following.
   i. Barr body   a. Trypsin
   ii. Nucleolar organiser   b. Lymphocytic culture

iii. G-banding
iv. Karyotyping
v. Chalones

c. Meiosis
d. Cell division
e. AgNOR-banding
f. Sex chromotion

9. Which of the following statements are true/false (T/F).
   a. Anaphase precedes metaphase.
   b. Prophase is the longest in both mitosis and meiosis.
   c. Daughter cells number is four in mitosis and does not resemble the parent cell.
   d. Reduction division is not essential during gametogenesis.
   e. Synthesis of DNA occurs during short interphase of second meiotic division.

4

Molecular Genetics

DNA ORGANIZATION OF CHROMOSOMES

Each chromosome is made up of coiled filaments of nucleic acid, the DNA (Fig. 4.1), surrounded by a covering of basic proteins called histones. A little amount of acidic protein is also present. The histones and DNA are collectively known as nucleoproteins.

Each somatic cell nucleus contains 5.6×10^{-12} gm of DNA. The double helix model of DNA structure, given by Watson and Crick in 1953, opened a new window on the molecular

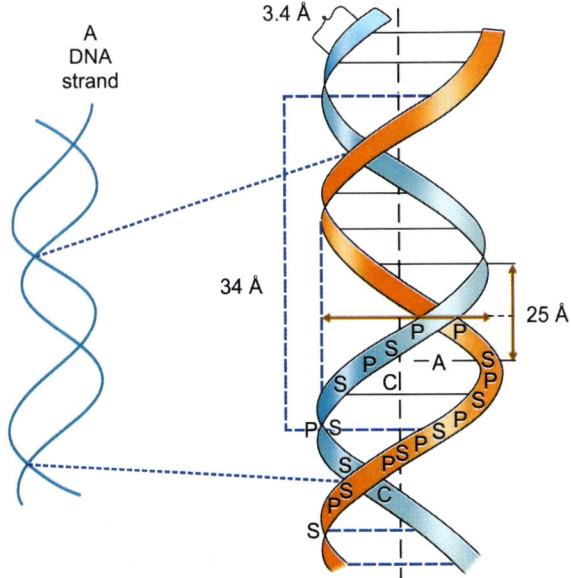

Fig. 4.1: DNA helix (25 Å in diameter)

A
DNA
strand

3.4 Å

34 Å

25 Å

organization of living system. Two strands of DNA molecule—a polymer of nucleotides formed from nucleosides which, in turn, is formed by nucleic acid bases are arranged in a helical manner with a maximum diameter of 25 Å and length of 3.4 Å between two base pairs and completing one turn in a length of 34 Å. The total length of DNA strand in a nucleus is 170 cm and in a single chromosome, when fully extended to the maximum is 7 cm.

Nucleosome: This term is used to denote the first coil or double helix (DNA) strand in the form of a cylinder about 8×11 nm in size. It contains about 146–165 base pairs of DNA strand wound round a histone core containing two molecules each of four histones (H2A, H2B, H3, and H4) inside, the DNA is situated on the outside. The two nucleosomes are joined to each other by linker DNA of about 35–60 base pairs. Five nucleosomes constitute one kilo-base (kb containing 1000 base pairs). One gene consists of 75 nucleosome of 15 kb length DNA. One chromosome on an average contains 6.5×10^{-6} gm nucleosomes and the nucleus of each cell contains 30×10^{-6} gm nucleosomes (Fig. 4.2).

Chromatin fibre: The term denotes the next level of coil producing a superhelix of 25 nm or 250 Å in diameter. It contains nucleosome with histone and ions, calcium and magnesium. The DNA here also is outside (Fig. 4.3).

Chromomere or band: It denotes the next higher package when the chromatin fibre forms a loop in repeated manner, and each loop is about 0.5 m in length and the loops are formed along a single axis. These long chromatin fibres are complexed with specific non-histone protein and divalent cations to produce chromosomes with highly differentiated segments along the whole length (Fig. 4.4).

About half the DNA in a chromosome at a time is made available to interact with external molecules, thus there will be only localized uncoiling along the length of chromosome for replication and transcription. During the metaphase stage of cell division which is the highest level of packing, the genes are no longer able to replicate and they can move freely without any harm to them.

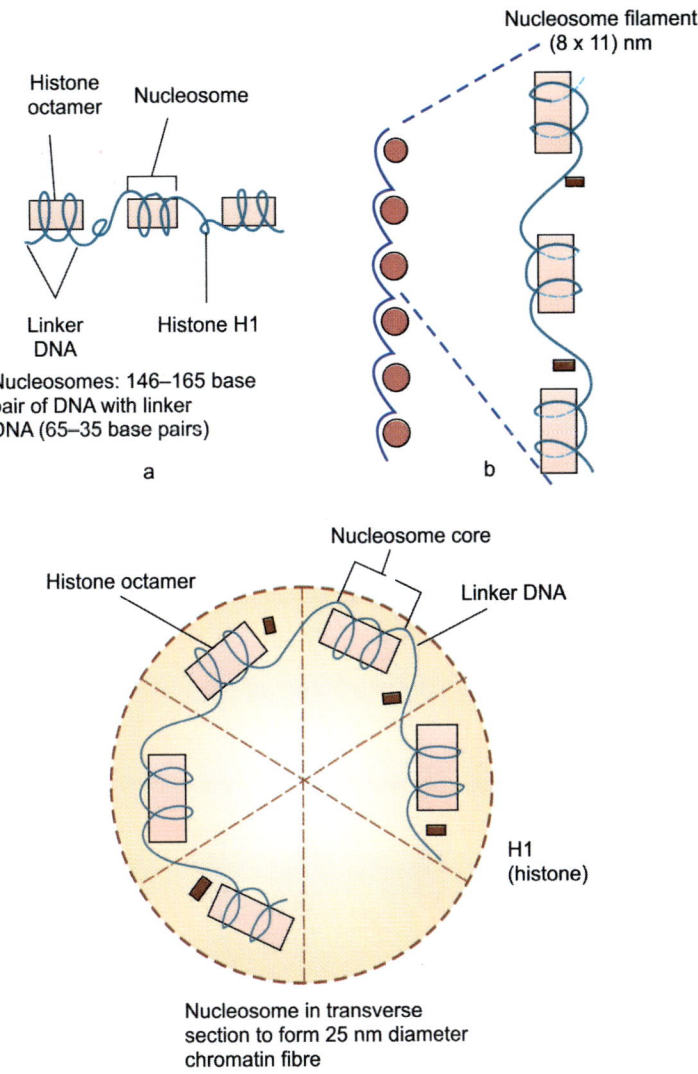

Fig. 4.2: Structure of nucleosome

MOLECULAR STRUCTURE OF NUCLEIC ACIDS (DNA AND RNA)

The nucleic acids DNA and RNA are chemically formed of two different types of bases—purines and pyrimidines (Fig. 4.5).

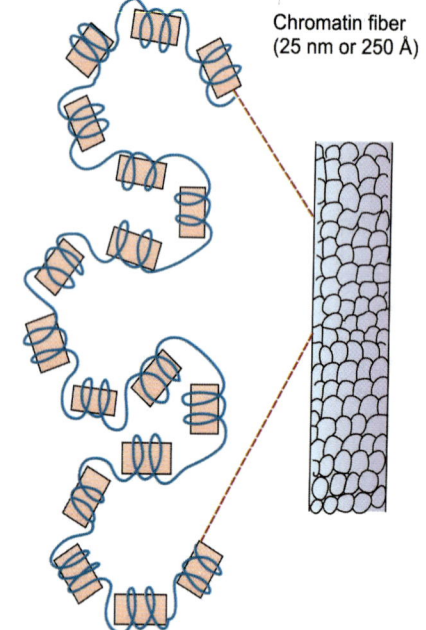

Fig. 4.3: Chromatin fibre of 250 Å diameter

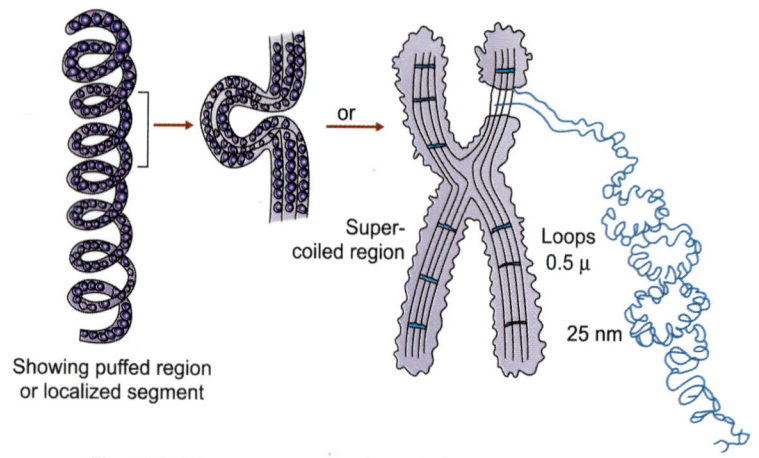

Fig. 4.4: Chromomere or band (super coiled region)

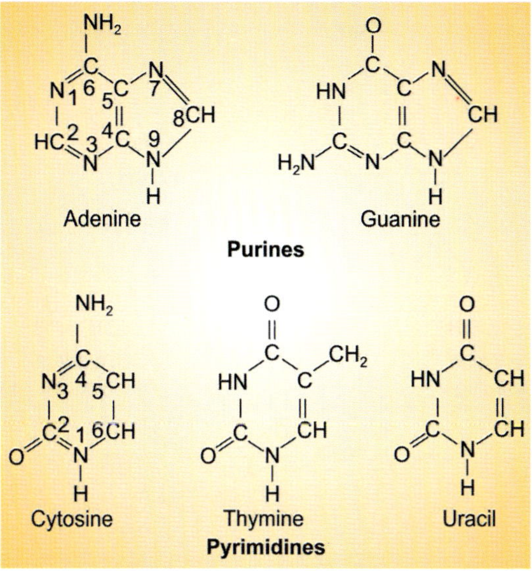

Fig. 4.5: Chemical structures of purines and pyrimidines

In DNA, the common purines are adenine and guanine, and pyrimidines are cytosine and thymine. The RNA contains uracil in place of thymine (methyluracil). Both carry coded information which can be translated to direct the activities of each cell.

Each molecule of DNA (arranged in two parallel strands wound spirally to constitute a double helix) can be simulated to a spiral ladder, the sides of which are formed of sugar and phosphate, and each stair is made up of a pair of nitrogenous bases, purines or pyrimidines. The chemical linkage between the base and pentose sugar is at the carbon atom of position 1 of sugar and nitrogen atom of pyrimidine at position 1 and in purine at position 9. The resulting molecule called nucleoside (Fig. 4.6) can act as an elementary precursor for DNA and RNA synthesis. When a nucleoside is linked with a phosphate group to form a nucleotide, which is capable of being included in the DNA or RNA molecule (Fig. 4.7).

Depending upon the number of phosphate group attached to the molecule it can be called as adenosine monophosphate (AMP) (Fig. 4.8), diphosphate (ADP) and triphosphate (ATP)

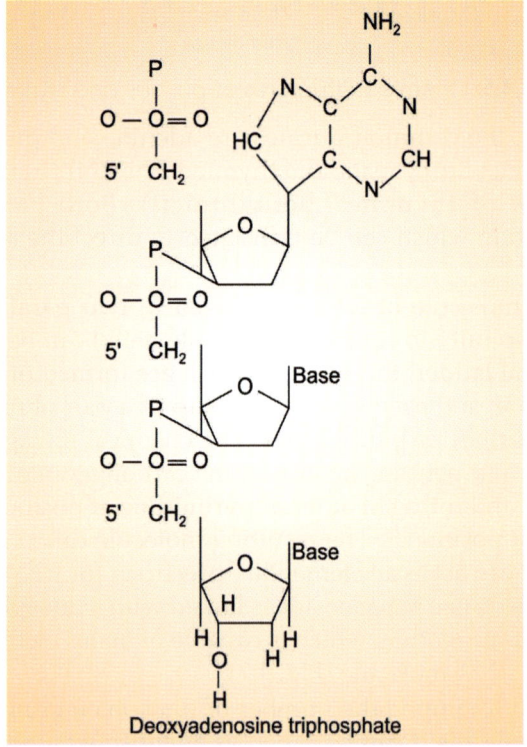

Fig. 4.6: Nucleoside

Fig. 4.7: Nucleotide or nucleic acid

(Figs 4.7 and 4.8). It is ATP nucleotide which acts as a precursor for DNA and RNA synthesis.

Two, three, a few or many nucleotides are joined together by only one phosphate group of ATP precursor for polymer and can be named as dinucleotide, trinucleotide, oligonucleotide, and polynucleotide respectively. This phosphate group bound to the 5' carbon of the pentose sugar on one nucleotide gets chemically bound to the 3' carbon of sugar of a second nucleotide and thus a series of 5'–3' phosphate linkages (Fig. 4.9) bind the nucleotides together. The phosphate bonds are covalent bonds and thus very strong. Polynucleotides are

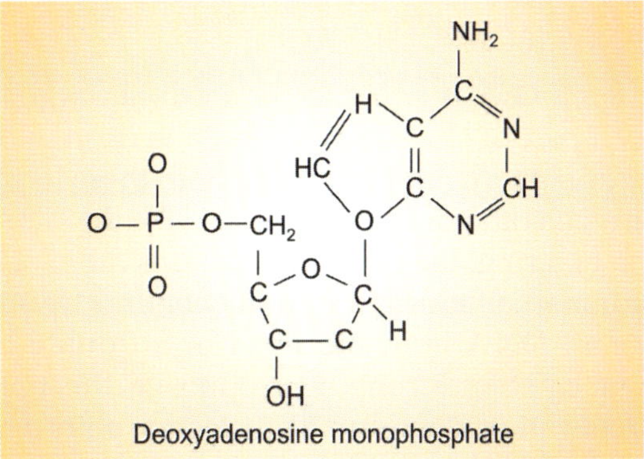

Deoxyadenosine monophosphate

Fig. 4.8: Deoxyadenosine monophosphate

Base pairs in DNA

Thymine   Adenine   Cytosine   Guanine
a   b

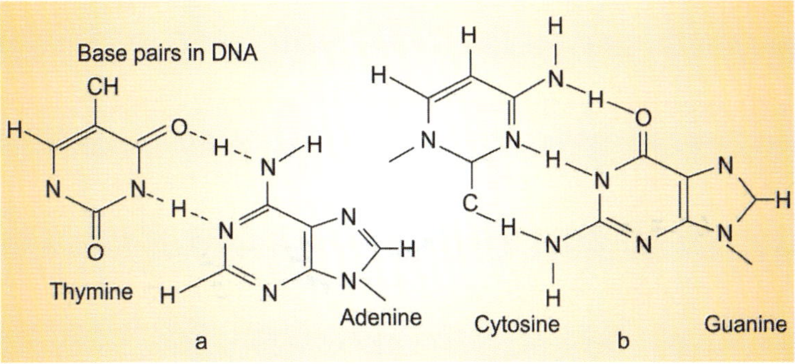

Fig. 4.9: Base pairing in DNA

structurally polarized, i.e. the two ends, one of 3' hydroxyl and other of 5' phosphate can be identified in a chain.

The bases of polynucleotide are situated at a distance of 3.4 Å in a double helix. Strands are oriented in opposite direction in such a manner that the 3' hydroxyl–5' phosphate end of one strand is opposed to 5' phosphate 3' hydroxyl end of other. The strands are held together by hydrogen bonds between bases in such a manner that base adenine always links with (Fig. 4.10) thymine and cytosine links with guanine in a DNA molecule. This complementary base pairing is obligatory. The replication of DNA molecule can occur only by splitting of strands forming two new complementary strands.

DNA (DEOXYRIBONUCLEIC ACID)

DNA can be found at two sites in a cell, in large amount in nucleus as a part of chromosome and a very small amount in cytoplasm as a part of mitochondria. Both these forms of DNA differ from each other in certain details, like the DNA thread is in the form of a ring, the nitrogenous bases differ and they are mainly of maternal in origin in mitochondral DNA while the chromosomal DNA is in the form of a double helix with complementary strands running in opposite direction for quick and fidel replication. There are 10 nucleotide pairs per complete turn of the double chain.

The replication is making a copy of DNA. This takes place during 'S' phase of interphase taking about seven hours before

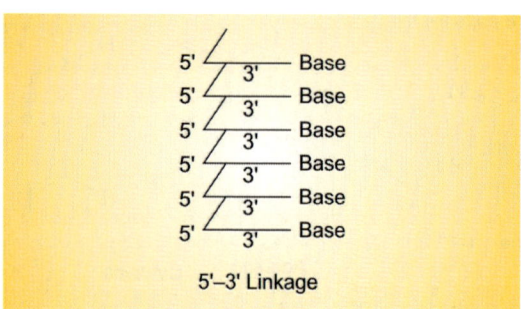

Fig. 4.10: Base pairing in DNA

the onset of mitosis or meiosis. Thus during replication (Fig. 4.11):

i. Two strands of DNA helix separate out.

ii. Each strand acts as a template.

iii. Each template forms a complementary strand.

iv. One template with its complementary strand forms a new DNA molecule.

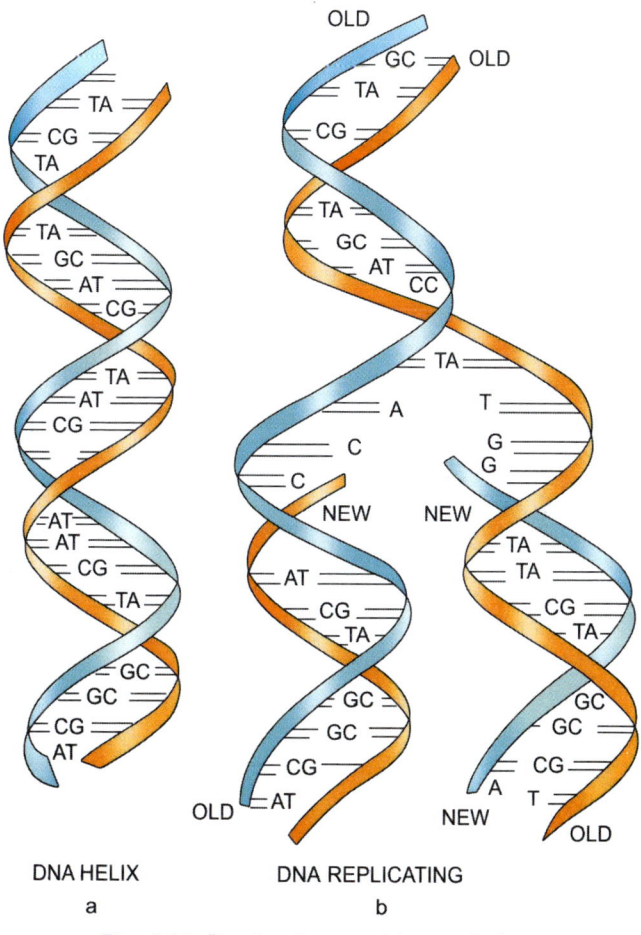

Fig. 4.11: Replication and transcription

CHROMOSOMAL DNA

Recent knowledge reveals that most of DNA in chromosome is in the inactive form, but it is packed in such manner so as to be easily available. Equal amounts of DNA and a protein–histone complex combine in a chromosome. A human diploid cell nucleus contains about 6×10^9 µm base pairs of DNA and 3000 base pairs are present in a length of 1 micron, the total length of DNA per nucleus is 2×10^6 µm, i.e. 2 meters, while nucleus itself is not more than 10 µm in diameter. The human genome contains about 2.7×10^9 µm nucleotide pairs which can code for about three million genes. Out of these, only 30,000 structural genes are formed by transcription and translation. The function of remainder of DNA is not known.

The secondary constrictions of the five pairs of acrocentric chromosomes carry the genes for 18S and 28S ribosomal RNA. These are nucleolar organiser and the cause of frequent non-dysjunction. Abnormalities in these chromosomes are still obscure. The gene for synthesis of 5S ribosomal RNA is situated near the ends of longer chromosomes.

Two classes of nuclear DNA have been described.

i. Unique with non-repetitive sequence DNA constituting 60–70% of genome. This is the structural gene. It also transcripts heterogenous RNA and precursor of transfer and ribosomal RNA.

ii. Repetitive sequences are present mainly in Q and G bands and it is presumed that in man most of the abnormalities in large chromosomes occur with large amount of such moderately repetitive sequences.

Classification of DNA

i. Nuclear DNA
- With repetitive sequence
- With non-repetitive sequence of genes.

ii. Mitochondrial DNA
- Responsible for cytoplasmic inheritance and it is present in a ring form and during cell division, is able to multiply independently.

iii. Recombinant DNA
- It is manufactured new hybrid form of DNA of wild origin, produced by inserting a gene or part of gene from one organism into genome of another organism to get a desired sequence of DNA.

RNA

RNA consists of a single strand of pentose sugar, ribose, phosphate, purine and pyrimidine bases. The pyrimidine base thymine is replaced by uracil, giving adenine–uracil base pairing and cytosin–guanine base pairing.

Classification of RNA

There are four types of RNA:
  i. *Messenger RNA:* Produced in nucleus, passes out through nuclear membrane to cytoplasm and dictates the amino acid sequence to be incorporated into a polypeptide chain.
 ii. *Transfer RNA:* Also known as soluble RNA (remaining in suspension following centrifugation) or adaptor RNA because of its structure, brings the amino acids from the cytoplasm to the required places along mRNA template. Each amino acid requires an activating enzyme to recognise the specific sites on amino acid molecule and tRNA. The anticodon of tRNA reads a specific codon on mRNA chain, thus placing the tRNA amino acid complex on correct site of mRNA.
iii. *Ribosomal RNA:* Present in ribosomes consisting of equal amounts of protein and non-specific RNA (rRNA). This is concerned with reading the code on mRNA and then bringing the tRNA–amino acid complex in line at the appropriate codon. This takes about 10 sec. Ribosomal enzymes form peptide bonds between amino acids and thus breaking off the polypeptide from its ribosome. A single mRNA can have several ribosomes attached to it at a time.
 iv. *Heterogenous RNA (HnRNA):* It is present in the nucleus and is probably the precursor of mRNA.

GENE AND GENETIC CODE

Gene is the theoretical unit of inheritance. Chemically it is a segment of DNA molecule responsible for the synthesis of a particular polypeptide. There are about one lakh genes in each human cell. This genetic constitution of an individual is the genotype of that individual. Genome is the term used to denote the full set of genes in an individual. The expression of these genes in the form of physical, biochemical or physiological traits or characters is the phenotype of an individual. A gene has the following properties.

  i. It is able to determine the character or trait, e.g. temperament, blood group, colour of skin, etc.
 ii. It is able to reproduce its exact replica (replication, Fig. 4.11).
iii. It can undergo mutation.

Each gene has a specific site on the chromosome to which it belongs. This is called as *gene locus*. The total number of genes present in a nucleus are derived half from one parent and other half from another parent.

Genes can be described to be having varying forms as follows:

  i. *Structural gene (cistron):* It controls the structure of a polypeptide comprising the protein.
 ii. *Operator gene:* It controls the adjacent structural genes and along with it is called as operon. It allows the transcription of structural gene only when not repressed.
iii. *Regulatory gene:* It controls the particular activity of a specific gene by exerting a negative control over protein synthesis by coding for repressers. It inhibits protein synthesis.
 iv. *Super gene (polycistron):* It is a group of genes which are responsible for coding of a number of functionally related proteins.
  v. *Architectural gene:* It controls the exact localization of enzymes and proteins in various cellular organelles.
 vi. *Temporal gene:* It regulates the protein synthesis in relation to time.

vii. *Pleiotropic gene:* A gene having more than one expression or trait phenotypically, e.g. gene responsible for phenylketonuria also results in other abnormalities like mental retardation and short stature, etc. This phenomenon of multiple expression is called as pleiotropism.

viii. *Sex linked genes:* Genes located only on sex chromosomes and concerned with the expression of sexual features. Most of these genes are located on the X-chromosome. Few Y-linked genes known as holandric genes have also been found out, e.g. hairy pinna.

ix. *Jumping gene:* Fixed locus of a gene on chromosome was the one of the central dogma. The changes of site can be either due to mutation or recombination. This has been shown in bacteria and Drosophila that the genes or even the segments of chromosomes move between and on chromosomes with as high a frequency as 10^2 Hz. Such genes are named as jumping genes. Such genes may possibly play a role in the change of normal cell into a cancer cell, or even speeding up the evolutionary process.

x. *Split gene:* The segments of DNA strands coding for a protein are separated by segments of strand that do not code for protein. So in eukaryotes, the concept that in a single gene, there are silent regions usually five or more, the effect of which never appears in the final gene product meaning thereby that a gene is split. The silent regions are called inserts or introns and functioning regions as exons or extrons. The length of one intron ranges from 10–10,000 bases. The introns are thought to be the frozen remnants of history or the sites of future evolution. The exon–intron concept may serve to solve many genetic problems like mutations, recombinations. The precise role of introns is not clear but can be summarized as follows:

a. The concept of introns regulating the turning off or on of genes is being discarded.

b. Introns act as structural genes or cistrons.

c. During evolution, if a cell has acquired a redundant DNA, intron is a simple device for discarding it.

d. Introns are ways to give diversity in gene sequence and thus providing an organism the selective advantage.

xi. *Overlapping genes:* Each gene is not a separate entity always, the separate genes can use same DNA sequence for protein synthesis using different coding frames. Thus it was observed that:

a. One gene can code for two different proteins.

b. One protein is coded in part by one gene in part by another gene.

c. The termination codon for one gene is the initiation codon for next adjacent gene. Such genes are called overlapping genes and obviously these are space saving device in minute organisms, where the DNA quantity is less as compared to the number of proteins required.

GENETIC CODE

The synthesis of proteins is directed by DNA, by specifically selecting the molecules made up of amino acids arranged in a specific linear sequence for a specific protein. There are twenty essential amino acids and only four nitrogenous bases for DNA. DNA should provide a code for each amino acid, thus three bases successively specifying one amino acid with possible number of combinations as 64 is the ultimate genetic code and triplet of bases is called as codon. Thus, the characteristics of a genetic code (Table 4.1) are:

i. It is universal in nature with few exceptions.

ii. It is triplet, i.e. three bases can code for one amino acid.

iii. There are no space between specific codons of a gene.

iv. There is no overlapping of bases.

v. Certain combinations of bases act as initiators and other terminators of gene, e.g. ATT, ATC, ACT or UAA, UAG, UGA code for the termination of a gene meaning that the synthesis of a polypeptide chain stops when these codons are read. The codon TAC, AUG codes for methionine and also initiates a gene, thus playing a dual role as seen in Table 4.1 of genetic code.

Table 4.1 : Genetic code to show the triplet (codon) of bases for messenger RNA and complementary DNA to code for a specific amino acid

| 1st base | | 2nd base | | | | | | | | | | | 3rd base |
1st base mRNA U	Aminoacid (AA)	DNA A	mRNA C	(AA)	DNA G	mRNA A	(AA)	DNA T	mRNA G	(AA)	DNA C	Base DNA
U for RNA or A for DNA	UUU	Phenylalanine	AAA	UCU	Serine	AGA	UAU	Tyrosine	ATA	UGU	Cysteine	ACA	U or A
	UUC	Phenylalanine	AAG	UCC	Serine	AGG	UAC	Tyrosine	ATG	UGC	Cysteine	ACG	C or G
	UUA	Leucine	AAT	UCA	Serine	AGT	UAA	Stop*	ATT	UGA	Stop*	ACT	A or T
	UUG	Leucine	AAC	UCG	Serine	AGC	UAG	Stop*	ATC	UGG	Tryptophan	ACC	G or C
C for RNA or G for DNA	CUU	Leucine	GAA	CCU	Proline	GGA	CAU	Histidine	GTA	CGU	Arginine	GCA	U or A
	CUC	Leucine	GAG	CCC	Proline	GGG	CAC	Histidine	GTG	CGC	Arginine	GCG	C or G
	CUA	Leucine	GAT	CCA	Proline	GGT	CAA	Glutamine	GTT	CGA	Arginine	GCT	A or T
	CUG	Leucine	GAC	CCG	Proline	GGC	CAG	Glutamine	GTC	CGG	Arginine	GCC	G or C
A for RNA or T for DNA	AUU	Isoleucine	TAA	ACU	Threonine	TGA	AAU	Asparagine	TTA	AGU	Serine	TCA	U or A
	AUC	Isoleucine	TAG	ACC	Threonine	TGG	AAC	Asparagine	TTG	AGC	Serine	TCG	C or G
	AUA	Isoleucine	TAT	ACA	Threonine	TGT	AAA	Lysine	TTT	AGA	Arginine	TCT	A or T
	AUG	Methionine**	TAC	ACG	Threonine	TGC	AAG	Lysine	TTC	AGG	Arginine	TCC	G or C
G for RNA or C for DNA	GUU	Valine	CAA	GCU	Alanine	CGA	GAU	Aspartic acid	CTA	GGU	Glycine	CCA	U or A
	GUC	Valine	CAG	GCC	Alanine	CGG	GAC	Aspartic acid	CTG	GGC	Glycine	CCG	C or G
	GUA	Valine	CAT	GCA	Alanine	CGT	GAA	Glutamic acid	CTT	GGA	Glycine	CCT	A or T
	GUG	Valine	CAC	GCG	Alanine	CGC	GAG	Glutamic acid	CTC	GGG	Glycine	CCC	G or C

*Chain termination ** Chain initiation

vi. The code is highly degenerate, meaning that most amino acids are specified by more than one codon because there are only 20 amino acids and 64 possible triplets.

vii. The chain is elongated with the formation of peptide bonding, and thus breaking up of amino acid–tRNA complex, setting free the tRNA to unite with another activated amino acid.

viii. The polypeptide moleculer being thus formed, get detached from the mRNA strand.

ix. The time taken by a ribosome to reach a terminator codon at the end of one gene is approximately 10 sec. After getting separated from mRNA, the tRNA becomes available to induce the formation of another polypepide.

Genetic Control on Protein Biosynthesis

It is a known fact that the protein synthesis is controlled by genes and external environment. There is a great amount of variability seen when the gene effect is concerned due to interaction with other genes and the environmental factors. The frequency with which a particular gene produce its effect in an individual is termed as its *penetrance* and the degree of effect produced by a specific gene is termed its *expressivity*.

The widely accepted operon concept says that a group of closely related structural genes are (cistrons) activated by an operator gene situated near it. Collectively both these genes known as operon, is controlled by two more segments of DNA, named as regulator and promotor genes which may or may not be near the operon. A regulator gene via mRNA strand synthesises a represser protein—1st order messengers, i.e. repressers, which makes them unable to repress the operator gene, which then become active. The promotor gene, initiates the structural gene for transcription, by becoming attached to the RNA polymerase (Figs 4.12 to 4.14). It controls the rate of mRNA synthesis of a known operon. All this work has been done in bacteria, giving underlying basis of present knowledge of protein synthesis.

Thus central dogma is unidirectional, i.e.

DNA → transcription → RNA → translation → proteins.

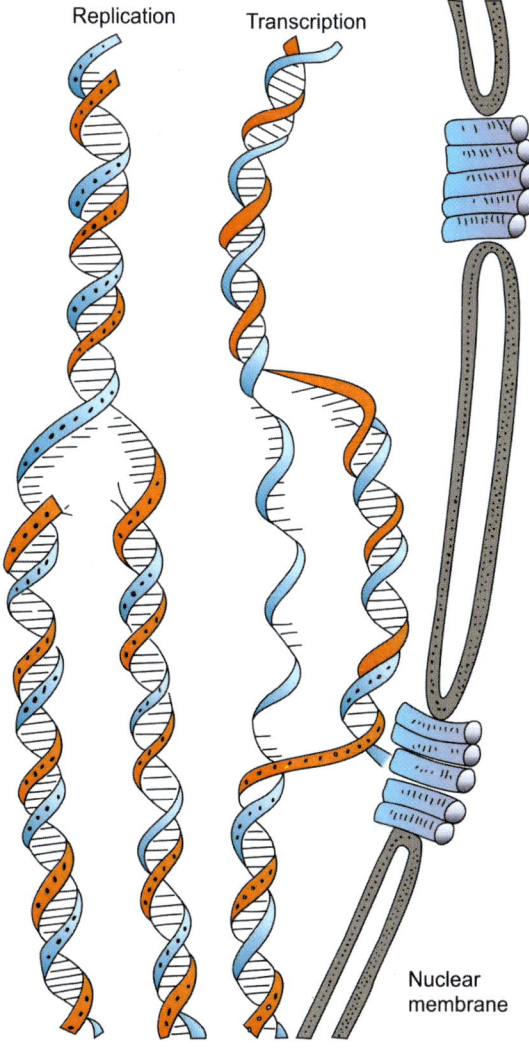

Replication   Transcription

Nuclear
membrane

Fig. 4.12: Replication and transcription

Contrary to central dogma, it has been recently found by viral studies that genetic information can also flow in a reverse direction, i.e. from RNA to DNA after RNA directed DNA synthesis. This is an important factor during embryonic differentiation and possible during carcinogenesis.

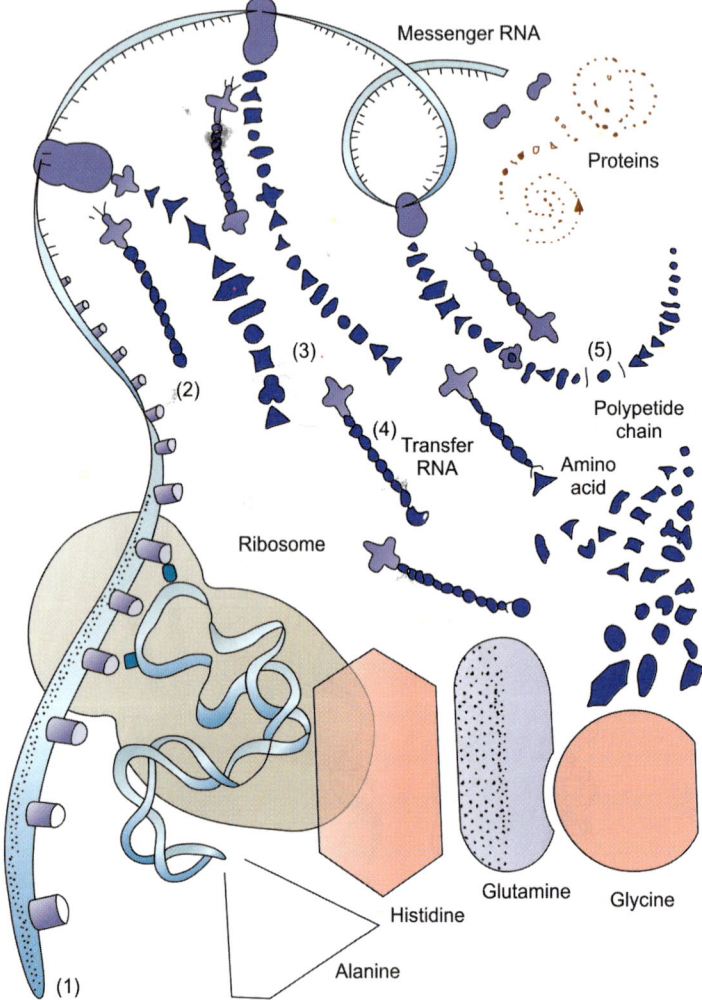

Messenger RNA

Proteins

(3)

(5)

(2)

(4) Transfer
RNA

Polypetide
chain

Amino
acid

Ribosome

Glutamine   Glycine

Histidine

Alanine

(1)

Fig. 4.13: Diagrammatic representation of the steps involved in the synthesis of protein

Detailed Gene Structure

The various lengths of DNA strands are named as follows:

Recon: It is the smallest segment of DNA strand, usually not more than two pairs of nucleotides which can be inter-changeable through genetic recombination.

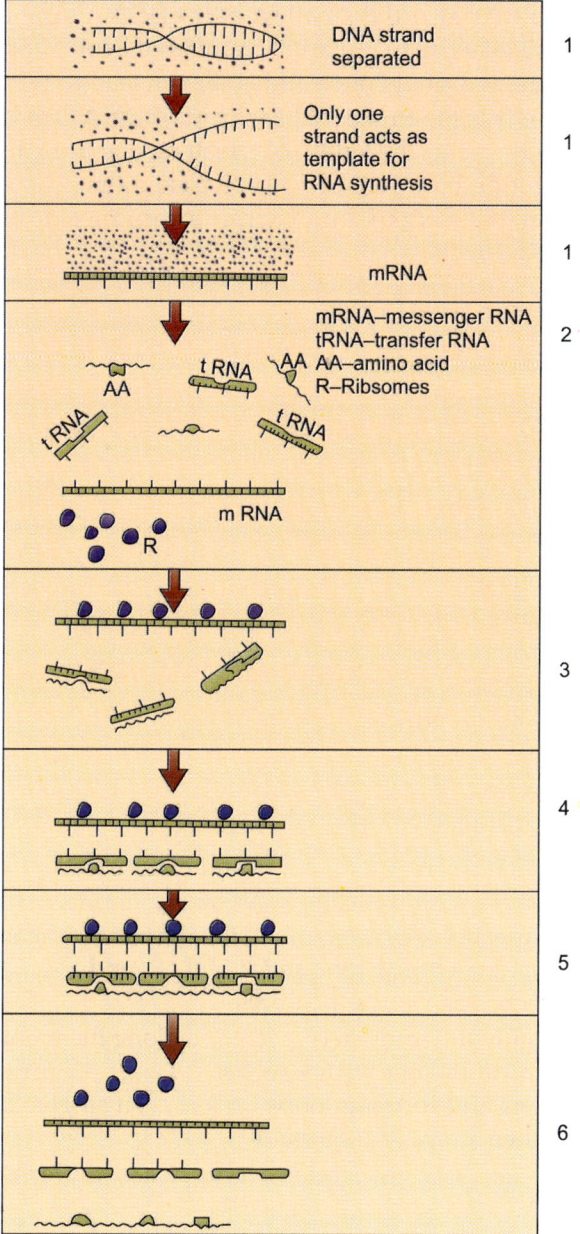

Fig. 4.14: Steps of protein synthesis

Muton: It is also the smallest part of DNA strand, when altered can give rise to mutation, i.e. altered expression of trait. The change in a single nucleotide pair can lead to mutation.

Cistron: It is the functional segment of DNA strand and in real sense the gene, the length of which ranges from more than 100 nucleotide base pairs to 30,000 base pairs. There can be more than 100 mutons in a cistron to produce a detectable phenotypic effect.

EXERCISE

1. Write short notes on:
   a. Nucleoproteins
   b. Nucleosome
   c. DNA
   d. Genetic code
2. Define:
   a. Recon
   b. Muton
   c. Cistron
   d. Nucleotides
   e. Chromotin fibre
   f. RNA
   g. Protein biosynthesis
3. Fill in the blanks.
   a. The first coil of .... strand in the form of .... about 8 × 11 nm is called ....
   b. A superhelix of .... Å diameter is containing .... with histone and .... and .... ions is known as .... fibres.
   c. A highly differentiated .... along the whole length of chromosome with specific .... protein and cations and forming loops .... a single .... is called .... or band.
   d. The .... nucleotide acts as .... for DNA and RNA.

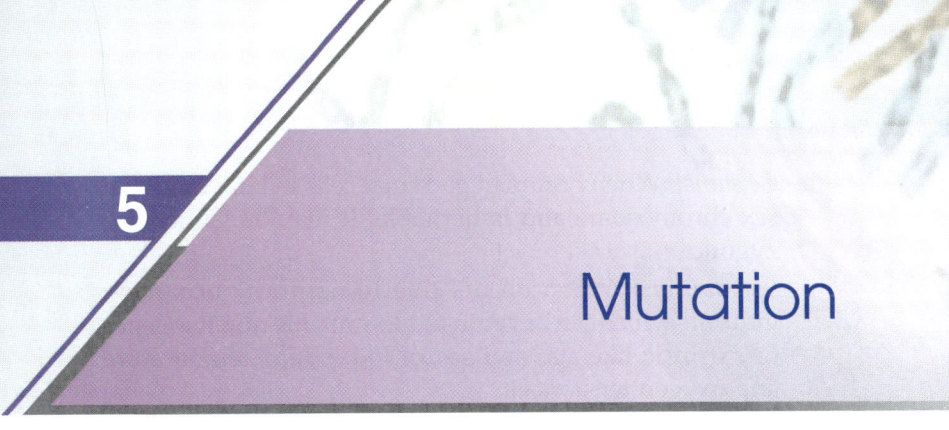

5

Mutation

SALTATIONS, SPORTS, DISCONTINUOUS VARIATIONS OR POINT MUTATIONS

The term mutation is defined as a physicochemical change in the gene, large or small, but not due to Mendelian segregation or recombination, leading to change in the expression of gene, in the form of remarkable deviation from the normal parental gene expression. Mutations may be large and conspicuous macromutations, small and inconspicuous micromutations. The latter is more common and is the main raw material constituting the evolutionary changes in plants and animals. Mutations can occur naturally in all animals and plants but can be induced artificially by exposing them to X-rays and chemicals known as mutagens. Mutant is the term to denote the resulting modified gene after mutation.

Classification

Mutations can be classified in various ways but broadly into
  i. Gene mutation
 ii. Chromosomal mutation or aberration, and
iii. Genomatic mutation or heteroploidy.

GENE MUTATION

Based on the phenotypic expression, genes can be further subdivided into:
  i. *Somatic:* When occurs in somatic cells, in autosomes or sex chromosomes—it is a rare event. Some cancers may be due to this but are not heritable.

ii. *Germinal:* When occurs in germinal cells in both auto and sex chromosome and is heritable. It may be gametic or zygotic.

iii. *Spontaneous:* When occurs due to naturally occurring inducers which can be intrinsic like mutable mutator genes or extrinsic like age and sex of individual, temperature and oxygen tension, etc.

iv. *Induced:* When induced experimentally by again intrinsic and extrinsic factors like X-rays, radium, ultraviolet rays, temperature, mustard gas, colchicine and some chemical mutagens like formaldehyde, hydrogen peroxide, urithane, phenol, caffaine, etc.

v. *Biochemical:* When there is a change in physiological and biochemical constitution of an individual due to mutation of a specific enzyme required for chemical reaction occurring during metabolism. This leads to metabolic disorder.

vi. *Spurious:* When mutations manifest only in offsprings as a result of crossing over.

vii. *Reverse:* When there is a reversion of mutation to normal.

viii. *Lethal:* When normal Mendelian expression is upset to cause death.

The most common mutagen in human beings is X-rays, and these rays can cause either immediate damage to the exposed individual or more insiduous damage to the genes in the reproductive cells affecting the future generations. The resultant mutations are generally proportional to the dosage of rays and the effect is cumulative. These mutations can be detected if they are of lethal type by CLB (cross over suppressor, lethal, Barr eye) experiment done in Dorsophila in the form marker gene.

CHROMOSOMAL MUTATION

The number and position of genes on a given chromosome are normally constant and fixed. A change in this number or position of one or both the genes of a pair in one or more chromosomes without any change in the total number of chromosomes is called as chromosomal mutation, or aberration or rearrangement. These mutations can be in the form of

i. Deletion or deficiency (including ring chromosome).

ii. Duplication including unequal crossing over.

iii. Inversion and insertion.

iv. Translocatlon—simple, reciprocal, Robertsonian, etc.

v. Position effect.

vi. Misdivision of centromere (isochromosomes).

The detailed explanation of the above forms is given in Chapter 6.

GENOMATIC MUTATION (HETEROPLOIDY)

The chromosomes occur in sets and the number of chromosome in man is 23 in haploid state, i.e. in gametes and 46 in somatic cells, i.e. in diploid state. Genomatic mutation means a variation from normal diploid number of chromosomes either in the form of variation in whole set known as euploidy or variation in total number, i.e. one chromosome less or more than 46, known as aneuploidy. Euploidy is further subdivided into:

Monoploidy: Seen in all gametes (normally as haploid in man).

Polyploidy: Triploidy or tetraploidy is uncommon in man being the mostly lethal and can be seen mostly in early abortuses.

Aneuploidy: When one chromosome is less or more can be seen in man and term is also applied when a segment of chromosome is less or more.

Euploidy does not cause genetic imbalance while in aneuploidy there is always such imbalance causing its effects. Aneuploidy can be hypoploidy called as Monosomy or nullisomy or hyperploidy called as trisomy or tetrasomy explained in Chapter 6.

EXERCISE

1. Define mutation.
2. Classify mutation.

3. Fill in the blanks.

    a. .... seen in all gametes.

    b. .... or .... mostly seen in early abortuses.

    c. When .... chromosome is less or more or even a
       .... of chromosome is less or more it is known as
       ....

    d. .... mutation is not heritable.

    e. .... does not cause imbalance, while ....
       always leads to imbalance in genetic material leading to
       its effects.

6

Abnormal Chromosome

The abnormal chromosomes carry the inherited abnormalities. The abnormal chromosomes can be studied under two main headings.

I. NUMERICAL ABNORMALITY

When there is abnormal number of chromosomes for a particular species, e.g. in human beings the number of chromosomes instead of being 46 shows a variation either in the form of multiples of haploid number. This is called *polyploidy*, diploid being the normal, triploid or tetraploid and so on being the abnormal number. Aneuploidy is the other form numerical abnormality where the exact multiple of haploid number is not there, e.g. 45 or 47 and so on, and this type of abnormality in number can be further subdivided into:

a. *Hyperploidy:* When there is addition of one or more chromosomes to the normal diploid number, e.g. trisomy $(2n + 1)$, i.e. 47 chromosomes, tetrasomy $(2n + 2)$, i.e. 48 chromosoms and so on.

b. *Hypoploidy:* When there is loss of one or more chromosome, e.g. monosomy $(2n - 1)$, i.e. 45 chromosomes, and nullisomy $(2n - 2)$ when both the chromosomes of a homologous pair are lost from the diploid set and chromosome number is reduced to 44.

Non-dysjunction

The term is used to denote when there is failure of two homologous chromosomes to separate during meiosis and resulting in one daughter cell having both chromosomes, the other daughter cell having none.

It can occur in autosomes and sex chromosomes during mitosis or meiosis. Autosomal non-dysjunction is less viable and one of the viable non-dysjunction of autosome of D and G group (Fig. 6.1) is Down's syndrome or Mongolism.

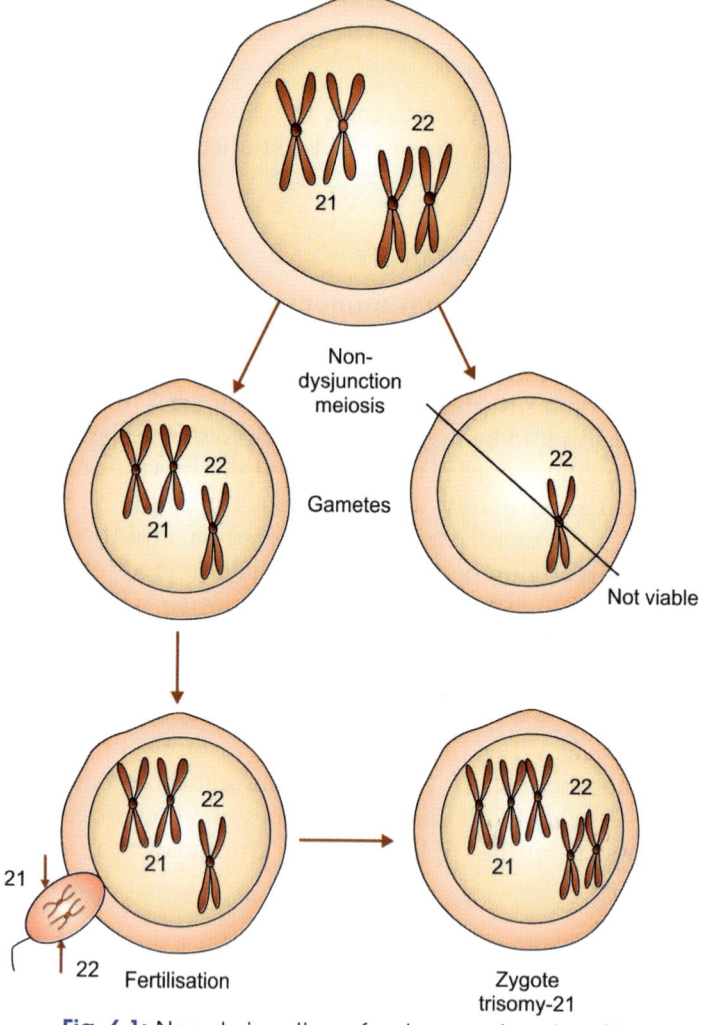

Fig. 6.1: Non-dysjunction of autosome (number 21)

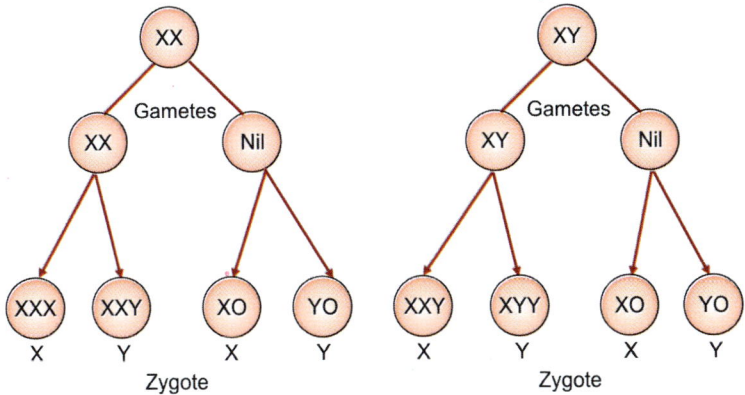

Fig. 6.2: Non-dysjunction of sex chromosomes

Non-dysjunction of sex chromosomes (Fig. 6.2) with significant effects phenotypically is seen in Turner and Klinefelter's syndromes. The abnormalities produced during meiosis is shown in Fig. 6.1, so that they can either remain in the same individual or pass to the progeny.

II. STRUCTURAL ABNORMALITY

When there is a change or variation in the arrangement of genetic material on chromosomes, i.e. different from the one normally seen. The cause of this is generally due to spontaneous breaks of chromosomes or these breaks are induced by some external factors like radiation, chemical or viruse, etc. It has been noticed that chromosomal breaks occur more frequently than the chromosomal abnormalities, i.e. the broken fragments usually unite to their original place leaving no trace of the break.

Symbols used to denote the chromosomal abnormalities in human beings:

1. Deletion — Del.
2. Terminal — ter.-peter-short arm terminal qter-long arm terminal
3. Short or upper arm of chromosome — p

4.	Long arm or lower arm of chromosome	q
5.	Duplication	dup.
6.	Isochromosome	i.
7.	Insertion	ins.
8.	Inversion	inv.
9.	Ring chromosomes	r.
10.	Satellite	Sat.
11.	Translocation	t.
	• reciprocal	rep.
	• Robertsonian	rob.
	• Tandem	tan.
12.	From To	13
13.	+ or – if placed before the chromosomes number means addition + or loss of chromosome as a whole, e.g. if placed after, denotes increase or decrease	±
	in the part of chromosome number, e.g. 5	p-
14.	Acentric	ace.
15.	Recombinant	rec.
16.	Secondary constriction	h.
17.	Tricentric	tri.
18.	Break	:
19.	Break and join	::
20.	Maternal	mat.
21.	Paternal	pat.

Normally majority of the chromosomal abnormalities are lethal either in early pregnancy or later and only a very small percentage of all such abnormalities reach to the stage of live births—a very good example of natural forces for quality control in human reproduction.

The numerical or structural abnormalities can occur at any time in any cell of body during one's lifetime. The abnormalities occurring in somatic cells will not affect the progeny, while the abnormality occurring in gonadal cells during gametogenesis will always pass to progeny and the resulting zygote will show the abnormality in all the cells. Such an individual becomes a carrier of the anamoly as the gametes are also abnormal and thus the progeny will show the abnormalities.

Structural abnormalities can be of following types.

i. ***Deletion or deficiency:*** When due to a break the terminal part of any arm of a chromosome is lost or deleted, it is known as *terminal deletion*. When there are two breaks again on one arm, the part between the breaks is deleted followed by the union of the sticky broken ends is known as *interstitial deletion*. The deleted portion lacking a centromere is normally lost during the subsequent cell division, unless the deleted fragment gets attached to the same or another chromosome (Fig. 6.3).

ii. ***Insertion:*** The broken segment of one chromosome gets translocated to another single break of another chromosome or in the position of two breaks leading to change in the order of genetics material but balanced (Fig. 6.4).

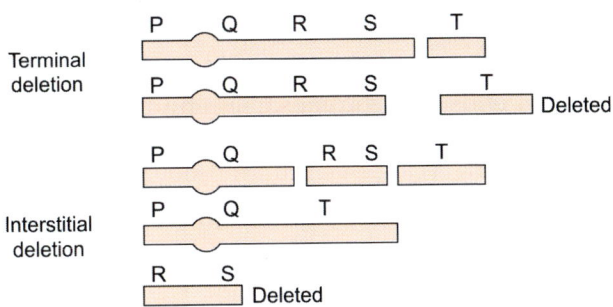

Fig. 6.3: Deletion

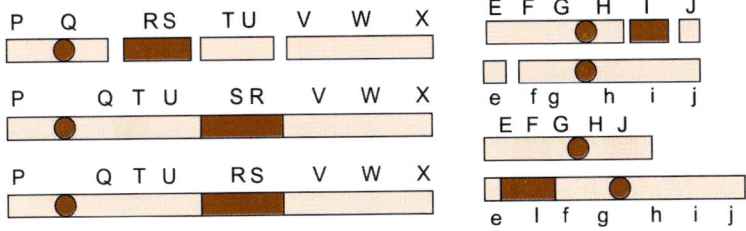

Fig. 6.4: Insertion

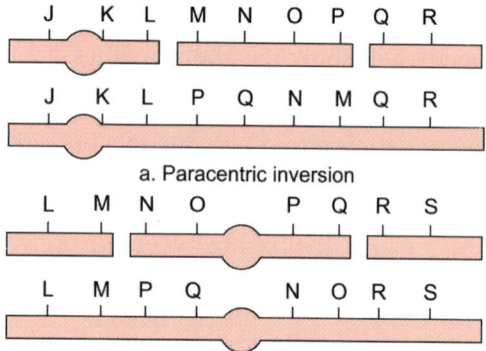

a. Paracentric inversion

b. Pericentric inversion

Fig. 6.5: Inversion

iii. ***Inversion:*** When after two breaks the segment rotates through 180° and gets reattached to same chromosome. It can include the centromere or may not include the centrotmere (paracentric or pericentric) (Figs 6.5a and b).

iv. ***Duplication:*** It may occur due to unequal crossing over or inversion or between X- and Y-chromosomes during gametogenesis (Fig. 6.6a and b).

v. ***Ring chromosomes:*** It is formed because of deletion of terminal ends of a chromosomes and broken pieces get lost while the other ends being sticky get attached to each other forming a ring. Such chromosomes are occasionally seen in humans (Fig. 6.7).

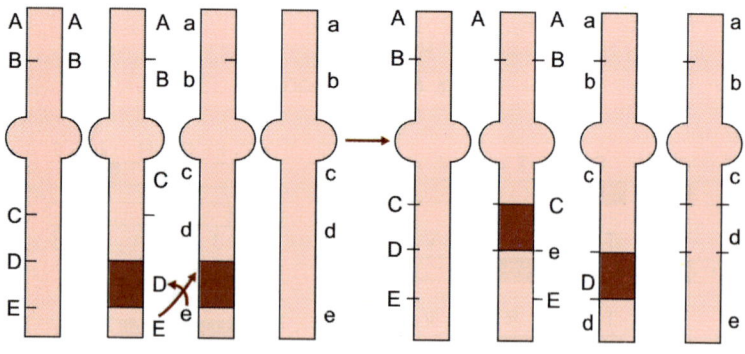

Fig. 6.6: Duplication in unequal crossing over

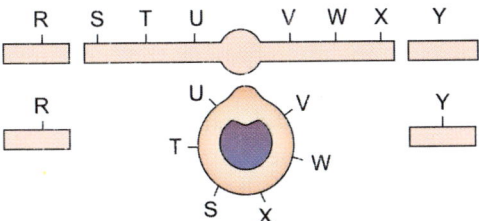

Fig. 6.7: Ring chromosomes

vi. *Isochromosomes:* It appears because of either separation of chromatids in such a manner that the short arms from one and long arms from another chromatid or there are breaks in short arm of one and long arm of another near the centromere and their broken ends uniting in such a manner that there will be duplication of the locus on the arms forming two different chromosomes (Fig. 6.8).

The results of these chromosomal deficiencies depend on the length and the role of the genetic material lost. In Dorsophila where minute deficiencies can be detected easily, deletion in some areas of a single chromosomere may be lethal, whereas, loss of even fifty chromomeres in other areas may be compatible with life depending upon whether the organism is homozygous or heterozygous for that deficiency. This proves that most of genes are

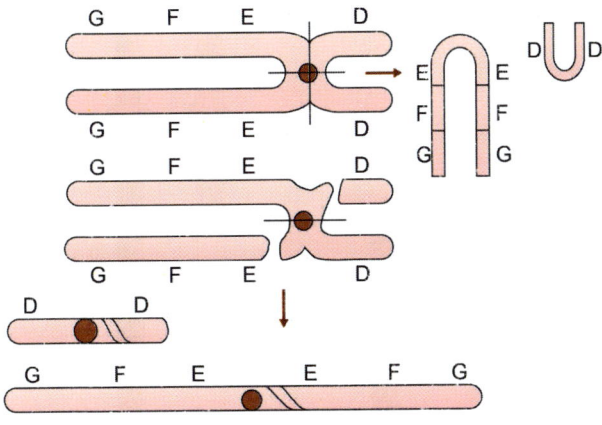

Fig. 6.8: Isochromosome

indispensable at least in a single dose for the development of a viable organism. In human, the common examples of deletion are seen in cri-du-chat, where short arm of chromosome No. 5 is deleted. Another example of loss of the whole chromosome in man, but compatible with life is absence of one X chromosome, called Turner's syndrome.

vii. *Translocation:* The most commonly observed abnormality (structural, Fig. 6.9) in a chromosome is a break at two places and the fragment gets attached to another chromosome—non-homologous forming a reciprocal translocation (Fig. 6.10). This is further divided into

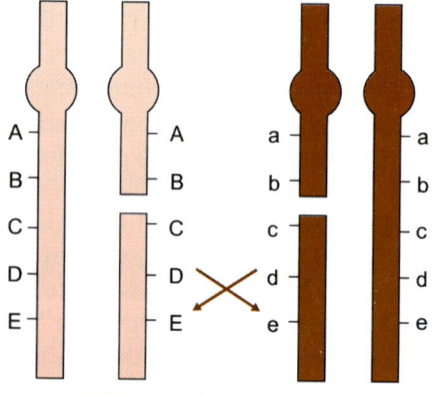

Fig. 6.9: Translocation

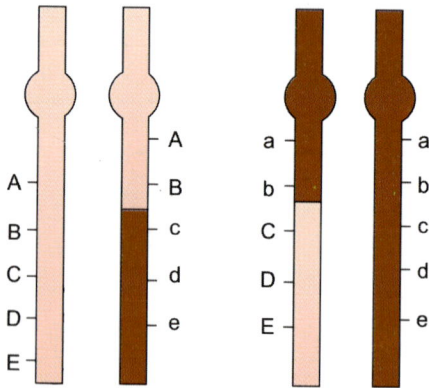

Fig. 6.10: Reciprocal translocation

homozygous when members of chromosomal pair exchange segments with another pair and heterozygous when only one member of each of both pairs exchange segments. In human beings, all such reciprocal translocations are heterozygous for the anamoly as one member of each pair has the normal sequence of arrangement and other member is involved in translocation. Since the genetic material present is normal in amount, such a heterozygous translocation is said to be balanced.

A translocation may not always give rise to an abnormal phenotype. However, the carriers of reciprocal translocation will show low fertility. During gametogenesis, the chiasma formation between the four members of a tetrad exhibit a characteristic pattern and it is due to random assortment that two thirds of the gametes of the reciprocal translocation carriers will have unbalanced genetic complement. The gametes formed will be in the proportion of one normal: one abnormal but balanced two abnormal and unbalanced combinations In: lAb (B): 2Ab (UB) (Figs 6.11a and b).

A simple translocation is exchange between different segments of same chromosome or another chromosome. This is an extremely a rare event.

The frequency of two break translocation leading to reciprocal translocation in living newborns is about two per thousand births.

Robertsonian Translocation

This is a special type of translocation known as centric fusion meaning thereby that there are two breaks near the centromeres of two acrocentric chromosomes involving in one short segment of short arm and long segment of long arm and unequal exchange between these arms leads to fusion between two long arms and another fusion between two short arms. Usually the short armed chromosome is lost. Centric fusion is a misnomer because it is actually a whole arm transfer rather than the fusion of centromeres. The pioneer work of Robertson on this type of translocation in grasshoppers and in many other animals

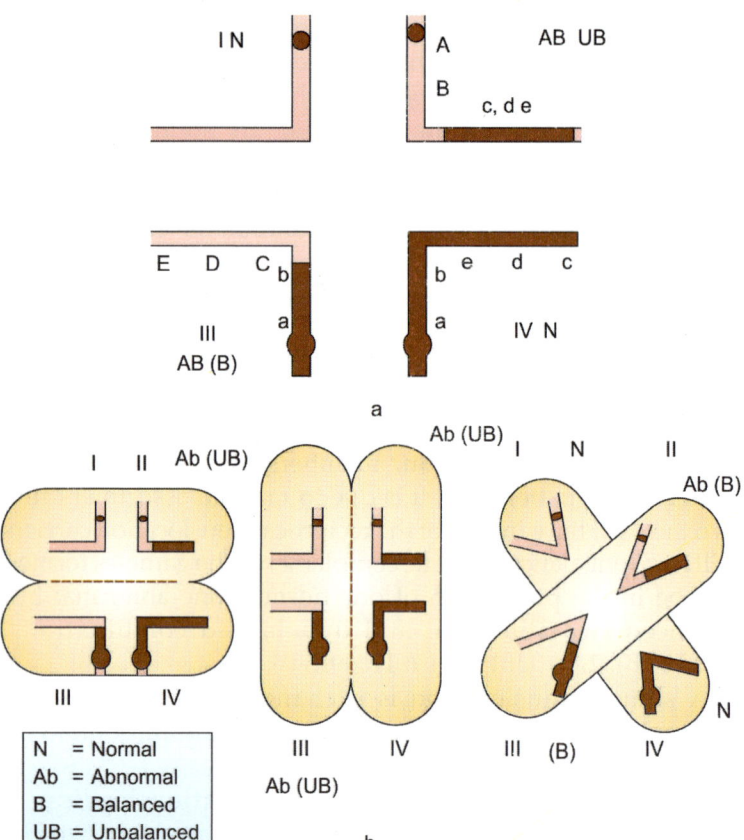

Fig. 6.11: (a) Tetrad of gametes in reciprocal translocation, (b) Gametogenesis in reciprocal translocation

was established, to serve during evolution the resulting differences in morphology and number of chromosomes (Fig. 6.12). In many organisations there is heterochomatin on both sides of centromere which is relatively inert and it tends to replicate later than the active euchromatin explaining thus the loss of short arm. The incidence of Robertsonian translocation in man is about 1 per 1000 births and it usually involves chromosomes No. 13 and 14 but 2% of all cases of Down's syndrome have Robertsonian translocation 14/21, 21/22 rarely 21/21. Thus a carrier of this translocation is

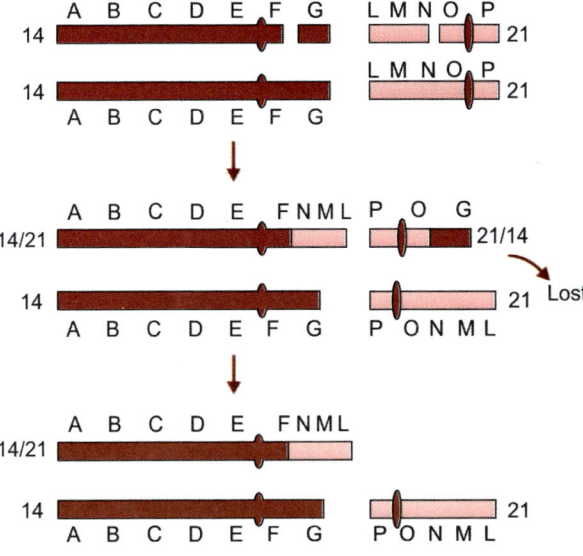

Fig. 6.12: Robertsonian translocation

phenotypically normal, being balanced as far as its genetic material is concerned. However during gametogenesis (Fig. 6.13) the imbalance results during meiosis, due to random segregations, 2/3 gametes tend to be abnormal leading to abortions and stillbirths. The remaining 1/3 gametes can produce viable progeny but half of them are the carriers of balanced Robertsonian translocation.

PHILADELPHIA CHROMOSOME

The karyotype in some chronic myeloid leukaemia patients (CML) discovered by Nowell and Hingerford, showed a chromosome was named as PHI chromosome (Fig. 6.14), establishing the first specific association between chromosomal aberation and cancer. It was not the simple deletion of long arm of chromosome number 22, but the deleted segment gets translocated to tip of long arm of chromosome number 9. The patients of CML, who lack the G-deletion also do not show the translocation at 9 q and patients are called as PHI negative. In 5% of PHI positive patients, the extra material can be found on

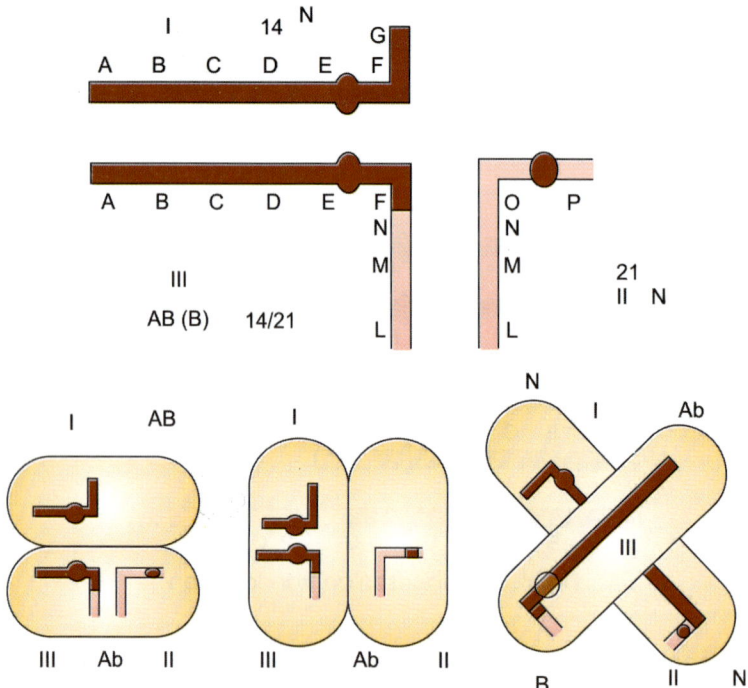

Fig. 6.13: Gametogenesis in Robertsonian translocation

other than number 9 and in 1% no extra material can be detected. About 85% of CML patients are PHI positive and are mosaics, i.e. all the body cells do not show PHI positive cells only bone marrow cells are PHI positive which appear in blood only during the acute stage or relapse of disease. This is still not clear that PHI is the cause or the effect of disease as the PHI anomaly is not present at the time of birth.

The effect of all these abnormalities can be seen during gametogenesis as shown in Figs 6.11, 6.13 and 6.15.

SISTER CHROMATID EXCHANGE (SCE)

Recently, it has been observed that during cell culture normally about 10 SCE occur per cell. With exposure to radiation or some carcinogens or mutagens in vitro, the number of SCE per cell increases.

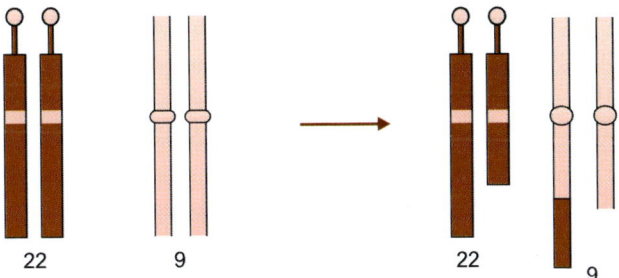

Fig. 6.14: Philadelphia chromosome

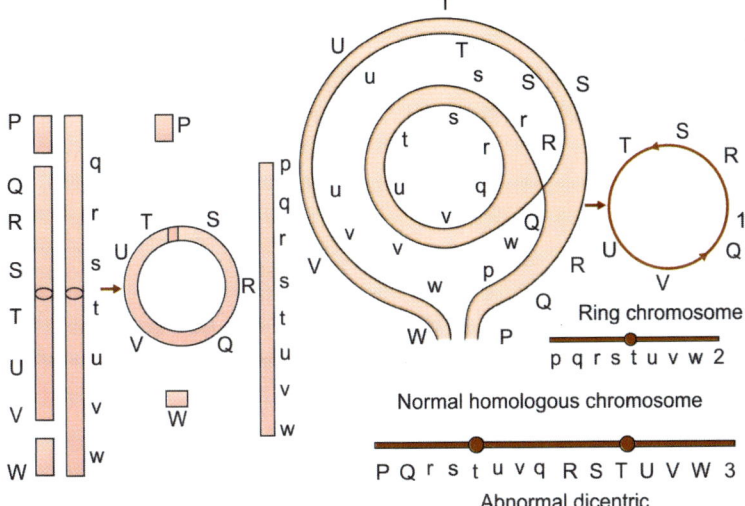

Fig. 6.15: Gametogenesis in ring chromosome

Abnormalities in chromosomes can be divided into:

i. Autosomal aberrations

ii. Sex chromosomal aberrations

These abnormalities manifest themselves in the form of some clinical syndromes involving a number of organs or systems, being interrelated with each other. The exact genetic and environmental factors leading to these aberrations are not known but predisposition of some factors has been well established.

The factors for chromosomal variations are:

a. Late age of parents for conception.
b. Genes predisposing to non-dysjunction.
c. Infections caused by viruses during pregnancy.
d. Exposure to radiation.
e. Autoimmune disease of parents.

In human the first clinical syndrome due to autosomal chromo-some aberrations has been described as Down's syndrome or mongolism, caused due to trisomy of chromosome 21. Later on, a number of other autosomal aberrations were described with characteristic features and the related syndromes are given in Table 6.1.

Table 6.1: Chromosomal aberrations and their significance

Chromosome No.	Syndrome	Clinical features
Chromosome 4 4p monosomy or trisomy 4q partial monosomy and trisomy	Apert's Carpenter's or Wolf's	In addition to growth and mental retardation, ocular hypertelorism, microcephaly, deformed ears, broad and beaked nose (acrocephalosynda-ctyly, craniosynostosis, midfacial hypoplasia)
Chromosome 5 during monosomy or trisomy of 5p	Cri-du-chat	Characteristic cat like cry, infancy, microcephaly, antimongoloid slant of the palpebral fissures.
Chromosome 13 trisomy	Patau's or Trisomy-D	Defects of eye, nose, lips and a holoprosencephaly with incomplete development of forebrain, olfactory and optic nerves. Polydactyly, narrow hyper-convex fingernails, skin defect in posterior scalp region are characteristic. Survival beyond a few weeks is unusual.
13q deletion or ring, trisomy or monosomy	13 long arm deletion	Microcephaly, trigonocephaly, micrognathia, large malformed ears, broad prominent nasal bridge, hyper-telorism, microphathalmus, hypoplastic or absent thumb and imperforate anus and perineal fistula.
Chromosome 18 18p monosomy or 18p or partial	Trisomy-E	Microstomia, short palpebral fissure, during clenching of hand, a tendency of 2nd over 3rd and 5th over 4th

Contd...

Table 6.1: Chromosomal aberrations and their significance (*Contd...*)

Chromosome No.	Syndrome	Clinical features
18q monosomy or 18q or trisomy		finger, a short sternum and characteristic low arched finger prints. Survival beyond few weeks is unusual. In 18q midfacial hypoplasia, microcephaly, atretic or narrow ear canal and prominent anti-helix of the auricle are main features.
Chromosomes—21-Trisomy or ring	Down's syndrome or Mongolism Trisomy-G	Flat faces with upward slant of the palpebral fissure, short hands, clinotic finger, palmar and solar prints occasionally affected, females reproduce this dominant inherited chromosomal abnormal.
21q	21 long arm deletion, Anti-mongolism	Antimongoloid faces, downslanting palpebral fissure, large malformed ears, microganthia, prominent nasal bridge, blephrochalasis, onchodysplasia, hypospadias, pyloric stenosis and thrombocytopenia.
22 ring chromosome	r(22) syndrome	Doe's eyes, low set eyebrows, anterior chamber maldevelopment, dental malformations, short stature, anal stenosis and myotonic dystrophy, etc.
Sex chromosomes XO	Turner's syndrome	Sex: female, short stature, ovarian dysgenesis, broad chest with widely spaced nipples, congenital lymphoedema, low posterior hair line, short neck and congenital heart. Mosaicism is very common and may modify the clinical involvement.
XXX, XXXX, XXXXX	X polysomy	Sex: female, severe mental growth retardation, patent ductus arteriosus, palpebral fissure slanted upward, small hands with clinodactyly of fifth finger are seen.
XXY	Klinefelter's syndrome	Sex: male, hypogonadism and gynae-comastia variants like XXXY or XXXXY are well known. The males are tall and psychopathic with aggressive behaviour.

EXERCISE

1. Define the following.
    a. Non-dysfunction
    b. Robertsonian translocation
    c. Philadelphia chromosome
    d. Ring chromosome
2. Fill in the blanks:
    a. .... abnormality in human beings can be either .... or ....
    b. Translocation can be .... or .... leading to the normal or .... phenotype.
    c. In human beings, trisomy of chromosome no .... leads to ....
    d. Cri-du-chat syndrome is due to .... of chromosome no ....
3. Write short notes on:
    a. Klinefelter's syndrome
    b. Turner's syndrome
    c. Down's syndrome
    d. Trisomy

7

Modes of Inheritance

INHERITANCE OF NORMAL MORPHOLOGICAL TRAITS

Much of the data on normal traits is uncritical. The difficulty in quantitative nature of these traits may improve by identifying the specific components of the normal variable trait.

The inheritance of normal physical features can not be classified into clear sharp demarcated modes of inheritance as per Mendelian's pedigree patterns. The typical examples of iris colour, thought to be simple as Mendelian inheritance is also variable because of many possible shades of colour. In general, genes for darker colour tend to be dominant to those for lighter colour, but a child born with darker iris than those of both parents is not necessarily the cause for divorce as the light iris may darken afer some months or even years of birth.

The innumerable shades of hair colour is of complex inheritance being governed by the environmental modification at least in some populations. The hair form or texture in the form of curly or straight is again complicated because of many degrees of waviness. Kinky hair is dominant inheritance in Caucasians and straight hair is dominant in Orientals but there is lack of critical data.

Baldness in old age is presumably a multifactorial inheritance, while pattern baldness before 30 years' age is a common trait to fit Mendelian's laws. it is caused by an autosomal gene which expresses iself in the heterozygote males only and not in females, presumably due to the presence of androgens, thus preventing the expression of gene in homozygous females.

Skin colour is again multifactorial showing intermediate dominance due to three different loci contributing to 18 possible shades of different amounts of melanin pigment. Little data is available for the red-skinned or yellow-skinned people.

Attached ear lobes is said to be recessively inherited but again in some individuals it becomes difficult to identify whether the lobe is attached or not.

Ear pits in the skin of ear lobes is of recessive inheritance. Tongue rolling ability is said to be dominant than inability to roll the tongue.

Handedness is definitely familial with variable frequency to resemble both the parents. This can be made to fit a single locus scheme if the right handedness or left handedness of heterozygotes is postulated as depending on subtle environmental variations.

Hand clasping and Hitch–hiker's thumb have no simple genetic basis though said to be recessive special ability to extend the terminal phalanx of thumb more than 30 degrees from the axis of first phalanx.

Dental anomalies, e.g. peg-shaped or missing lateral incisors is due to a dominant gene. Webbed toes of varying degrees found usually in females only in some families is said to be of autosomal dominant inheritance.

Physiological Variations

PTC taste threshold-ability to taste phenylthio carbamide or N-C-S group of goitrogenic chemicals is markedly variable. This striking physiological difference is determined by a single locus, i.e. the recessive nontaster allele. It is not related to taste acuity in general. The heterozygotes have higher threshold for PTC taste than the homozygous tasters. There is an evidence to suggest that the nontaster genotype predisposes the development of toxic goiter.

Ear wax: The type whether it is brown, wet, sticky or dry flaky grey in colour appears to be recessively inherited.

Colour blindness: For red or green (protanopia or deutanopia) is said to be X-linked inheritance seen in males.

Beetroot urine: Appearance of red pigment in urine after the intake of beetroot is due to an autosomal recessive gene inheritance.

Factors Leading to Variation in Expression of Genes

i. *Penetrance:* It means the ability of a gene to express phenotypically and inability is called as nonpenetrance. This ability in an individual remains as an all or none phenomenon, while in a population when some individuals do not express, the trait is said to have reduced penetrance.

ii. *Expressivity:* The phenotypic expression of an abnormal trait may not be of same degree in all the individuals having that gene. The expression is somewhere in between the two extremes of normal and abnormal.

These phenomena of penetrance and expressivity suggest that the phenotypic expression of genes depends at least partly upon some modifying genes.

iii. *Pleiotropy:* When a single gene is responsible for a number of distinct and unrelated phenotypic traits, leading to one gene several effects. Thus, many genetic defects forming a syndrome are the examples of pleiotropy.

iv. *Association and linkage:* Nonrandom occurrence of two phenotypically separate traits in a population, e.g. trait for blood group 'O' and peptic ulcer and duodenum show a significant association. As the hereditary basis of peptic ulcer is not established, it is very likely that some physiologic association and not the genetic linkage with blood group 'O' renders a person more susceptible to peptic ulcer. When the genes for two different traits are situated close to each other on the same chromosome, there are greater chances that the two genes will be transmitted together, contradicting Mendel's law of independent assortment, which has been found to be true only when genes under study are found to be situated on two different chromosomes.

MODES OF INHERITANCE OF ABNORMAL TRAITS

The inheritance of a genetic disorders (Table 7.1) can be due to:

i. A single gene defect
ii. A chromosomal defect
iii. A multifactorial defect

Table 7.1: Common dominantly inherited disorders

S.no.	Disorders
1.	Achondroplasia
2.	Anorectal anomalies (some types)
3.	Brachydactyly
4.	Cataracts
5.	Charcot–Marie–Tooth disease
6.	Clinodactyly
7.	Dentinogenesis imperfecta
8.	Ehlers–Danlos syndrome
9.	Haemangiomata
10.	Hernia: Inguinal, bilateral
11.	Huntington's chorea deformity
12.	Lentigines
13.	Marfan's syndrome
14.	Migraine (familial)
15.	Myotonic dystrophy
16.	Neurofibromatosis
17.	Osteogenesis imperfecta
18.	Polycystic kidneys
19.	Polydactyly
20.	Polyposis coll
21.	Retinitis pigmentosa
22.	Sickle cell traits
23.	Split-hand
24.	Syndactyly
25.	Tuberous sclerosis
26.	von Willebrand's disease
27.	Wardenburg's syndrome

i. A Single Gene Defect

In a homologous pair of autosomal chromosomes when only one member of a pair of gene is expressed, it is said to be dominant but when both the members of a pair of gene are expressed, it is said to be recessive. Therefore the inheritance can be of dominant or recessive type. Different genotype combinations can produce various phenotypes in medical genetics.

The patterns followed by a single gene trait within families over a number of generations can be recorded by a chart known

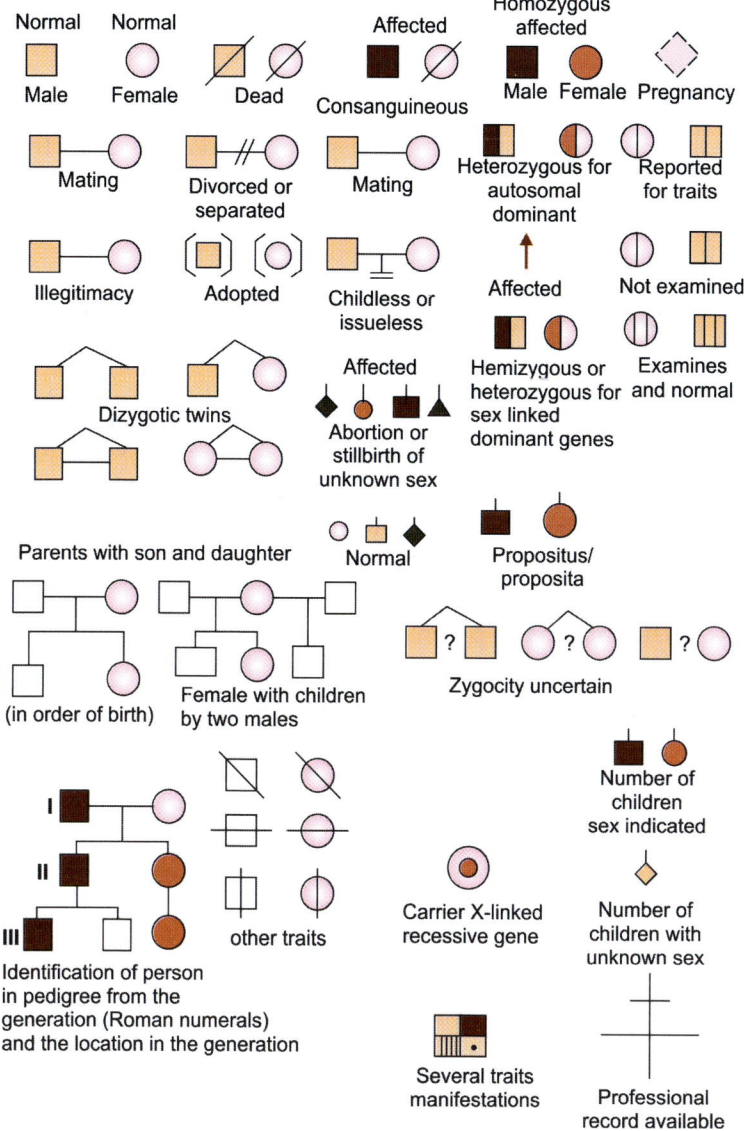

Fig. 7.1: Symbols used for pedigree chart

as *pedigree chart* which can be defined as a chart prepared by using internationally accepted symbols (Fig. 7.1) by taking family history from the patient known as index or proband case.

These single gene traits are determined by the following factors:

i. The chance distribution of gene responsible for a trait passed from parents to children through gametes.

ii. The gene determining the trait is autosomal or sex-linked.

iii. The gene for the trait is dominant or recessive.

iv. The factors affecting the expression of the trait of that particular gene, e.g. environment, penetrance, pleiotropy, heterogeneity, variability in expression and age of onset, partial or complete sex limitation, and interaction with two or more genes.

A. The common features of the *autosomal dominant* inherited traits are (Fig. 7.2):

1. The trait appears in every generation with no skipping.

2. On an average the trait is transmitted by an affected parent to half of the children born.

3. The unaffected parent does not transmit the trait to the offspring.

4. The sex of the child born is not influenced by the transmission or occurrence of trait.

The features of autosomal dominant traits commonly seen in human are:

a. *Dentinogenesis imperfecta with* 1:800 incidence, showing typical opalescent brown colour teeth and crown of teeth wear down easily.

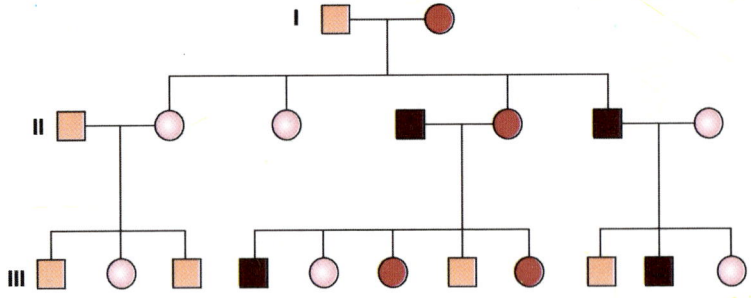

Fig. 7.2: Typical pedigree chart of autosomal dominant inheritance

Table 7.2: Common recessively inherited conditions	
S.no.	Conditions
1.	Adrenogenital syndrome
2.	Agammaglobulinaemia (some types)
3.	Albinism (complete form) (Tyrosinase –ve and +ve forms)
4.	Cystic fibrosis
5.	Deafness (some types)
6.	Glycogen storage diseases (including galactosemia)
7.	Laurence–Moon–Biedl syndrome
8.	Letterer–Siwe disease
9.	Microcephaly (some types),
10.	Microphthalmus
11.	Mucopolysaccharidoses (some types)
12.	Retinitis pigmentosa
13.	Sickle cell disease
14.	Spastic paraplegia
15.	Tay–Sachs disease
16.	Werdnig–Hoffmann disease

b. *Achondroplasia:* When the skeletal system is affected and the affected person is a short limbed dwarf with large head and bulging forehead, bridged nose and usually lethal in early infancy if present in homozygous form.

B. The common features of an *autosomal recessive* inherited traits are (Table 7.2):

1. There is consanguinous marriage between the parents of the affected individual.
2. The trait appears only in sibs and not in the parents, children or other relatives of the affected individuals.
3. The risk of recurrence is 1:4.
4. The trait can appear in any sex, i.e. both males and females are equally affected (Fig. 7.3).

The example of autosomal recessive trait are:

Laurence–Moon–Biedl–Bardlt syndrome with ulnar polydactyl and typical moon shaped faces.

Sex linked single gene disorders can be inherited from both Y-chromosome and X-chromosome by dominant or recessive genes. Since the genes present on sex chromosomes differ in

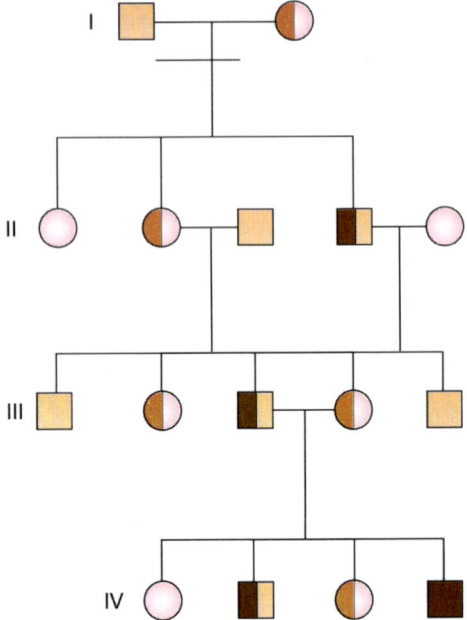

Fig. 7.3: Pedigree chart to show autosomal recessive inheritance

distribution in both sexes, the pattern of inheritance differs from that of autosomes. For practical purposes sex linked inheritance means X-linked, because the only Y-linked Mendalizing gene for hairy pinna and H-Y antigen are known at present.

C. The common features of an *X-linked dominant* trait are (Table 7.3):

i. The trait from affected males passes to all his daughters with all the sons normal.

ii. The trait in females if heterozygous is transmitted to half the number of children of either sex. The females if homozygous for the trait, transmits it to all the children thus transmission being similar to that of autosomal dominant inheritance.

iii. The females are affected twice more than males depending on whether the female partner is heterozygous or homozygous for the trait. It also depends on whether an

Table 7.3: Common X-linked disorders

S.no.	Disorders
1.	Agammaglobulinaemia (Bruton) + Swiss types
2.	*Albinism, Ocular
3.	Aldrich syndrome
4.	Cleft plate (some types)
5.	*Colour blindness
6.	Diabetes insipidus
7.	Ectodermal dysplasia
8.	*Ehlers–Danlos syndrome (type V)
9.	Fabry's disease
10.	Glucose-6-phosphate dehydrogenase deficiency (variants African type or A-minus)
11.	Glycogen storage disease (type VIII)
12.	Gonandal dysgenesis (female type)
13.	Haemophilia A
14.	Haemophilia B (Christmas/diseases)
15.	Hydrocephalus (aqueductal stenosis)
16.	Hypophosphataemic rickets
17.	Icthyosis
18.	Incontinentia pigmenti
19.	Melnick-Needles (multiple malformations) syndrome
20.	*Microphthalmia
21.	Mucopolysaccharidosis (Hunter type 11)
22.	Muscular Dystrophy–Duchenne
23.	Muscular Dystrophy–Backer
24.	Spastic paraplegia syndrome
25.	Retinitis pigmentosa
26.	Telecanthus–hypospadias syndrome
27.	*Testicular feminisation
28.	Wildervanck's syndrome

*More frequent occurrence

affected person marries a normal or affected female as shown below:

a. Affected male marrying a normal female produces all affected heterozygous daughters, but normal sons (Fig. 7.4A).

b. Affected male marrying an affected homozygous female produces all children affected with daughters being homozygous and son hemizygous (Fig. 7.4B).

c. Affected male marrying an affected heterozygous female (consanquneus produces half affected homozygous daughters and half heterozygous affected daugthers and half affected hemizygous and half sons normal (Fig. 7.4C).

d. A normal male marrying an affected homozygous female produces all children affected with daughters heterozygous and sons hemizygous (Fig. 7.4D).

e. A normal male marrying an affected heterorygous female produces half the children affected of either sex heterozygous or hemizygous (Fig. 7.4E).

D. The common features of an *X-linked recessive* trait are (Figs 7.5 to 7.7):

1. Males are usually showing the trait being uncommon in females.

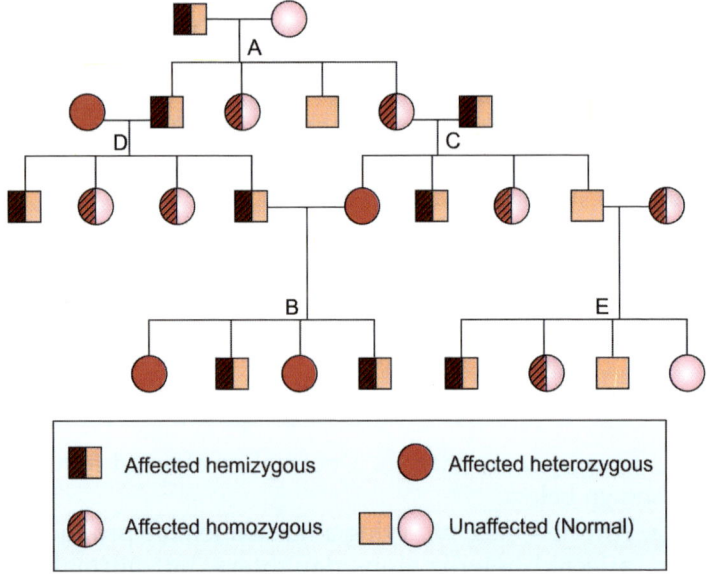

Fig. 7.4: Pedigree chart of X-linked dominant inheritance

2. The trait will pass from father through his daughters to all of his grandsons.
3. The trait requires a series of carrier females for transmission to males and thus the affected males are related to each other through females.

The X-linked dominant inheritance can be distinguished from autosomal dominant inheritance only by the sex of the affected offsprings of affected males as the affected homozygous female transmits the trait to all her children.

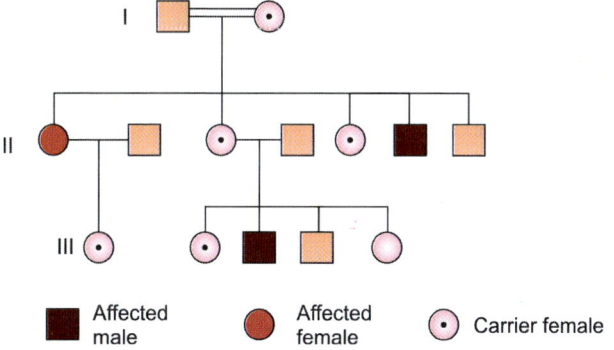

Fig. 7.5: Pedigree chart showing affected female in X–linked recessive disorder

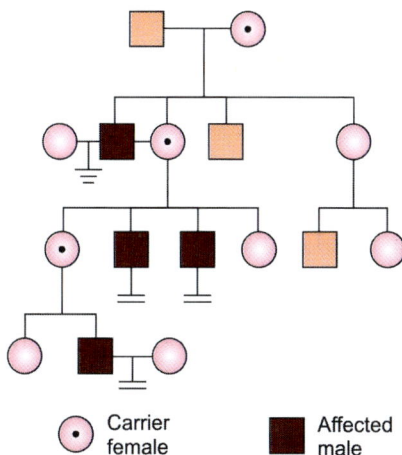

Fig. 7.6: Sketch showing affected males who cannot reproduce in X-linked recessive disorder

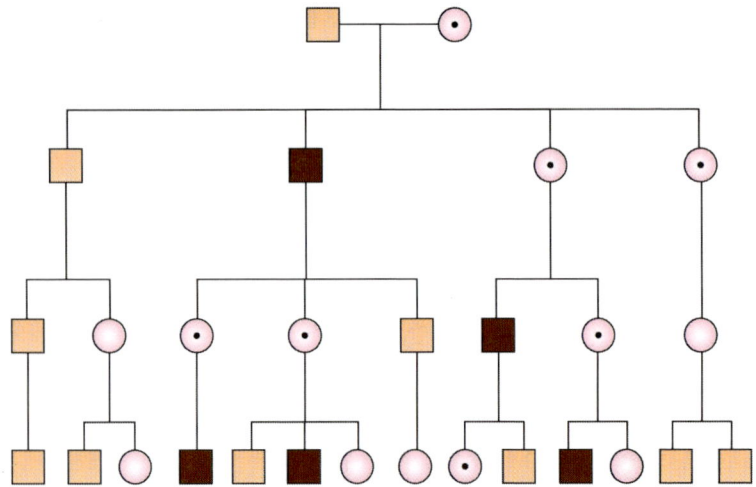

Fig. 7.7: Pedigree chart of X-linked recessive inheritance

E. The features of a *Y-linked inheritance* which is called as holandric are:
1. The traits of nonhomologous genes present in Y-chromosome are always seen only in males.
2. Affected males transmit the trait to all his sons and not to the daughters.
3. All the genes present on Y-chromosome are always expressed phenotypically as there is no homologous.

Y-chromosome but X-chromosome will have homologous nonhomologous regions.

ii. Chromosomal Defects

The various defects of autosomes as well as sex chromosomes have been described in chapter 6 and the transmission of defects from parents to offsprings will be detected if the gametes show the defect. The phenotypic effects of some chromosomal defects are shown in Table 6.1.

iii. Multifactorial Defects

These defects can be inherited because of following reasons or factors:

i. *Genetic Heterogeneity*

Genetic heterogeneity means a particular phenotype can be the result of a number of distinct genes instead of a single gene. This property of genes can be revealed by a detailed pedigree analysis. The examples of genetic heterogeneity are retinitis pigmentosa, which gives a pedigree chart of either A-linked or autosomal inheritance. Similarly the three main types of muscular dystrophy differ in their mode of inheritance, age of onset and severity. The explanation of congenital deafness in both parents with children having normal hearing is that the parental deafness is caused by different recessive genes and each parent has a normal allele at the locus for which the other has an abnormal gene. There are about 32 different genes inheriting various forms of deafness.

ii. *Sex Limited and Sex Influenced Genes*

The genes are present only on autosomes and not on X- or Y-chromosomes, but are expressed only in one sex, e.g. anatomical and physiological characteristics of the female sex such as age of onset of menarche, sexual features of a female pelvis or characteristics of male in the form of distribution of hair on body or type of growth of beard. Such traits genes are not concerned with determination of sex, being bipotential in a diploid set of chromosomes. However, there is a distinct sexual dimorphism, i.e. primary and secondary—sexual differences visible externally which are either present at birth or appear later in life. This explains that all cells have necessary genes to produce primary and secondary characters associated with both sexes, i.e. a female has all the genes for production of beard and a man has genes necessary for fully formed breasts but the potentialities of these genes do not get realized to express themselves. This can be due to stimulation of one set of gene and inhibition of another set of genes in opposite sexes. This simultaneous stimulation and inhibition, accomplished by various mechanisms like environment.

X- and Y-chromosomes, XO, ZW and honey bee methods are used for sex determination and differentiation.

The sexual dimorphism affects the penetrance and expressivity of some genes of autosomes not concerned with the sex determination. When a varying degree of expression of a genotype is seen in both the sexes, it is sex controlled, sex modified or sex influenced genetic expression. The common examples of such incomplete penetrance and variable expressivity in human being are hare lip, cleft palate and pattern baldness.

There is a great variability in the manifestations of a genetic trait, as regards the age of onset and its qualitative expression due to interaction of nonallelic genes. The age of onset varies from early embryonic life to late age, e.g. some chromosome aberrations are lethal and thus shows early abortion, some congenital abnormalities seen at birth like polydactyly, some genetic diseases manifested only when the child grows, like Tay-Sachs disease seen at four to six months, Duchenne muscular dystrophy when the child starts walking, and acute intermittent porphyria in young adult and Huntington's chorea manifests much later in life.

The interaction of nonallelic genes in a single gene trait is proved by the expression of different genetic traits in individuals having different genetic background, e.g. ABO secretor trait is produced by a pair, two gene pairs acting together to produce a phenotype. These individuals secrete the antigens A, B and H in saliva and thus has both genes A and Se.

iii. *Multiple Alleles*

When more than two different alleles are present at a given locus of a chromosome it is called as multiple allelism. Blood groups represent multiple allelism where all the alleles happen to be normal. There can be multiple allelism where one is normal and others are abnormal in dominant or recessive conditions. Duchenne muscular dystrophy is a disorder which is transmitted by a recessive gene situated on the X-chromosome. There are other variants of this disorder thought to be transmitted by a recessive gene situated on X-chromosome expressing as a mild or benign form of muscular dystrophy known as Becker type.

iv. *Polygenic Inheritance*

Many of the traits inherited, instead of being governed by a single gene, i.e. alleles at one locus, are determined by a number of genes, each having a minor effect in expression of a single trait. Such traits are called polygenic type or mode of inheritance is polygenic. The multifactorial term can be used as synonymous with polygenic but the trait is determined by multiple genetic and nongenetic environmental factors. Such traits are characterised by having continuous variation and manifest themselves with poorly defined traits as compared to sharply defined traits like black and white. Each gene contributes a minor affect in expression of that trait, resulting in quantitative variation in its manifestation in a population. Graphically this is shown as a Gaussian, bell-shaped or normal curve while recording the height of individual, pulse rate, IQ, refractive index, dermatographic ridge count, basal metabolism or length of fingers or weight of lungs, etc. in a population (Fig. 7.8).

The basic evolutionary material is the genes that determine the ordinary normal inherited differences between normal people, storing a vast reservoir of potential variability, enabling the species to adapt itself to different environments and also enabling it to change gradually and smoothly in response to changing external conditions.

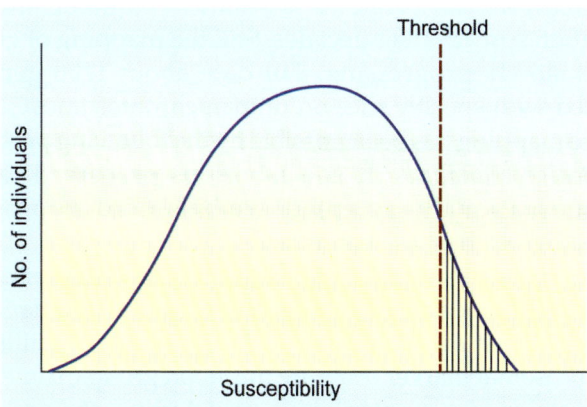

Fig. 7.8: Polygenic inheritance (Gaussian curve)

The basis of developmental defects is due to a quasi-continuous or threshold trait of polygenic nature. If the timing of development shows a continuous variation, extremely slow growth can lead to failure of normal development at a later stage, where punctual completion of this is vital. For example, if the ureteric bud of the mesonephric duct does not complete the development of the collecting tubule system on schedule, the kidney may become polycystic. The *threshold controlled liability concept* is to express specific phenotype, i.e. the susceptibility of normal distribution of a given trait is divided into normal and abnormal by a threshold. The example of this is pyloric stenosis. The incidence in general population with ratio in two sexes being 5:1 as far as males females are concerned. This accounts for different thresholds in two sexes for getting pyloric stenosis, i.e. in general population if the threshold for males is lower than that for females, more males than females will be suffering from the disease.

GENE LOCALIZATION OF INDIVIDUAL CHROMOSOMES

Chromosomal mapping is based on the methods which determine the linked loci of a chromosome (Table 7.4) known as linked genes and *synteny* means all the genes on a chromosome which do not assort independently.

The methods pertaining to study of linked genes in human is difficult as the progeny is small in number and each generation spreads over decades. Still the mapping of genes in man is slowly progressing. Till date about 1700 genes are specified with specific sites on human chromosomes.

Gene mapping has been possible by the following procedure:

i. *Pedigree analysis:* It is a laborious process. These are internationally accepted symbols used to prepare a pedigree chart as shown in Fig. 7.3.

ii. *Gene markers:* Autosomal and X-linked markers. These marker genes are quite frequent in general population and thus the studies can be done easily in some families. The autosomal marker traits are the blood groups, some serum proteins like hepatoglobins, transferrins, etc. and ability to taste PTC. The X-linked marker trait are colour

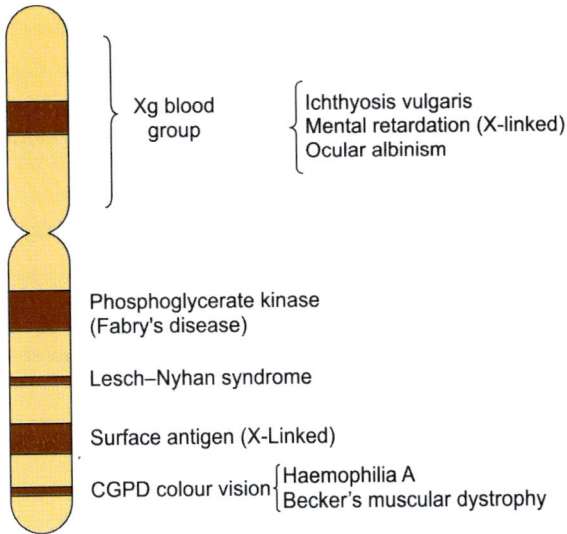

Fig. 7.9: Tentative map of the X-chromosome

blindness, Xg blood group and some cases of glucose-6-phosphate dehydrogenase deficiency (Fig. 7.9).

iii. *Study of a rare disorder* due to deletion of a part of chromosome—a method of expression because of loss of normal allele on deleted chromosome, e.g. deletion of short arm of chromosome 5 expressed as cri-du-chat syndrome characterised by mental retardation and underdeveloped larynx leading to a mewing cry of a child.

iv. *Study of linked genes and crossing over* by fusing the cells from two different species in the presence of a virus. The fused cell is then cultured and the hybrids are studied for the resulting chromosome constitution and chances of enzyme synthesis, e.g. an enzyme thymidine kinase can not be synthesized by the mouse cells, which are fused with human cells capable of synthesizing the enzyme. When all the human chromosomes are lost from the hybrid after some generations except chromosome number 17 and still the hybrid is able to synthesize the enzyme, proving thereby that the gene responsible to synthesize the enzyme is located on chromosome number 17 in man.

Table 7.4: Disorders located at a particular locus on various chromosomes

Chromosome no.	Various loci for disorders
1	Rhesus, elliptocytosis, congenital cataract, Duffy blood group, retinitis pigmentosa (dominant)
2	Red cell acid phosphatase-I (ACP1), aryl hydrocarbon hydroxylase
5	Hexosaminidase-B
6	Major histocompatibility complex (MHC—HLA), spinocerebellar ataxia (dominant), adrenogenital syndrome
7	Collagen (I) structural gene
9	ABO blood group nailpatella syndrome
15	Hexosaminidase-A
17	Thymidine kinase
19	Polio- and Echovirus sensitivity
20	Adenosine deaminase
21	Superoxide dismutase-1
Y	Y histocompatibility antigen
X	Xg blood group, G6PD, colour vision.

v. *Many bacteria synthesize* an enzyme group named endonucleases. These enzymes specially recognise the nucleotide sequence in DNA from any organism for a specific length of DNA (usually four to six nucleotides are recognised by one enzyme) and it is always at the same site by that particular enzyme. Thus these are named as restriction enzymes. These enzymes (more than about 100) have been isolated from various bacteria for commercial purposes. Such enzymes are now being used to locate the normal as well as genes producing disease on the chromosomes. The enzymes are also named as chemical scissors because the DNA is cut into restriction fragment length (RFL).

A number of genes have been localized on the autosomes and sex chromosomes thus making it possible to diagnose the genetic disorders in human beings. Recently, even mitochondrial genes have been located and their complete sequence has been mapped forming a genome and it has been found that these are responsible for neuropathic disorders.

The clinical application of mapping of chromosomes lies in detection of carriers (heterozygous), undiagnosed and/or unmanifested genetic disorders, and also prenatal diagnosis.

EXERCISE

1. Write short notes on:
   a. Penetrance
   b. Expressivity
   c. Pleiotropy
   d. Association and linkages.
2. Define pedigree chart. Draw a pedigree chart of autosomal dominant inheritance.
3. Write the common features of the following.
   a. Autosomal dominant inheritance
   b. Autosomal recessive inheritance
   c. X-linked dominant inheritance
   d. X-linked recessive inheritance.

8

Biochemical Genetics

INTRODUCTION

The understanding of the changes from the zygote to child phenotype can be achieved only after having a complete knowledge of biological interactions and parts played by heredity and environment on genes. For this understanding, the chemical structure of a gene with its position on DNA strand, and DNA–protein interaction and interdependence should be known. This knowledge forms the basis of phenomena like cell growth, differentiation, structural and metabolic transformations within cells, and individual variations in response to drugs. Since all proteins, whether structural or enzymatic, are inherited, any gene mutations are likely to be reflected in the altered structure or in the altered enzyme dependent metabolic function. The biochemical genetics will cover the following topics.

a. Inborn errors of metabolism
b. Blood groups
c. Haemoglobinopathies
d. Immunogenetics
e. Pharmacogenetics

Biochemical genetics is the study of genes governing biochemical processes involved during metabolism of various substances processed in the body. Garrod was the first scientist to give the idea that all metabolic processes in living organisms occurs in steps. Each step is governed by one enzyme. The 'one gene one enzyme' concept given by Beadle and Tatum (1941), proposes that each enzyme is coded by a specific gene so that a defect in gene will result in total or partial enzyme defect, which in turn leads to a metabolic block, producing pathologic consequences. The clinical manifestations are the result of disturbances brought about by the metabolic block which produces pathological effects because of the following metabolism:

   i. Accumulation of precursor just preceding the step where there is a block. This accumulated precursor itself can have toxic effects or with alternate minor pathways may lead to the production of toxic metabolites.
  ii. Stoppage of subsequent steps in the metabolism. Whenever a feedback mechanism is involved in the control of metabolism such deficiency would lead to overproduction of toxic metabolites by stimulating agents.

   The example of above factors are shown in Fig. 8.1 for phenyl-alanine metabolism.

A. INBORN ERRORS OF METABOLISM

When a specific enzyme defect produces a metabolic block to produce pathological symptoms, this is given the name of inborn errors of metabolism.

   These inborn errors of metabolism can be classified into:

   i. Disorders of amino acid metabolism, leading to diseases like phenylketonuria, leucinosis, alkaptonuria, albinism, homocystinuria, etc.
  ii. Disorders of carbohydrate metabolism, like galactosaemia, glycogen storage diseases (glucose-6-phosphatase deficiency), pentosuria etc.
 iii. Defects of purine and pyrimidine metabolism, like gout, juvenile hyperuricaemia and xanthiuria, etc.
  iv. Disorders of lipid metabolism (lipidosis) like Gaucher's, disease, Tay-Sachs disease, Niemann–Pick disease, essential hypercholesterolaemia, etc.
   v. Mucopolysaccharidosis like Hurlers' and Hunters' syndromes and fucosidosis, etc. There is accumulation of mucopolysaccharide in connective tissues due to defect in lysosomal enzyme.
  vi. Defects of mineral metabolism, like Wilson's disease. Haemochromatosis due to defective copper and its metabolism respectively.

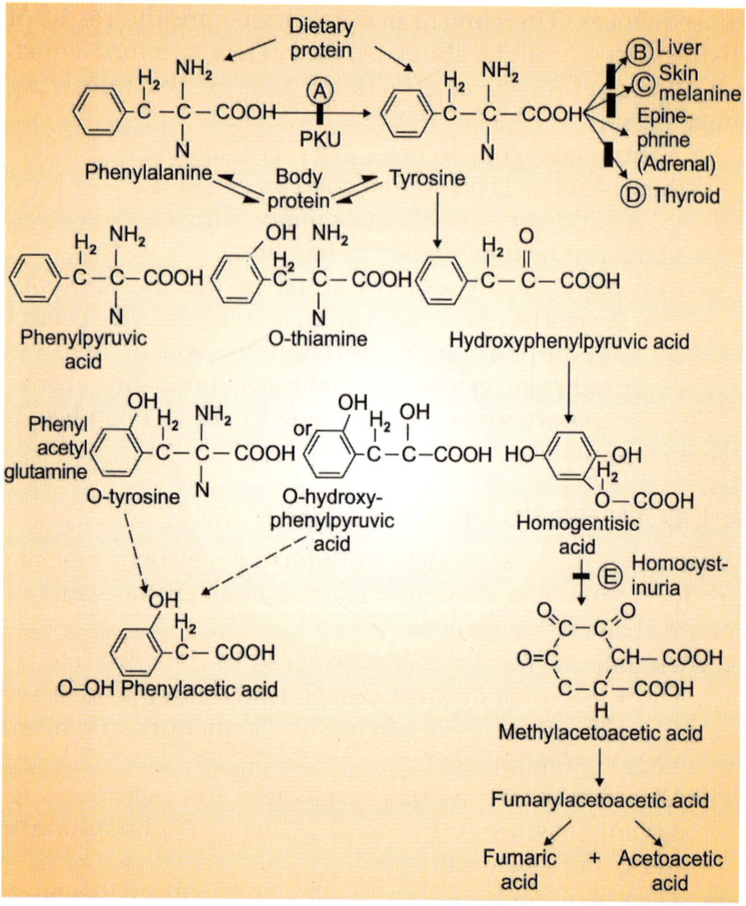

Fig. 8.1: Metabolic steps of phenylalanine and blocks at A, B, C, D, and E to produce various effects, (A) PKU, (B) oxidation (liver), (C) melanin (skin), (D) thyroxine (thyroid), (E) homocystinuria

vii. Defects in membrane transport—like renal glycosuria, glucose–galactose malabsorption, cystinuria, hartnup disease, phosphaturia, etc.

Selected inborn errors of metabolism are shown in Table 8.1 with defective enzymes, clinical manifestations, mode of inheritance, incidence, diagnostic methods and treatment.

Table 8.1: Inborn errors of metabolism

S. No.	Enzyme (Protein) defective	Disorder	Clinical manifestation	Mode of inheritance and zygosity	Incidence	Diagnosis	Treatment
1. Defects in Metabolism of Aminoacids							
(a) Phenylalanine	Phynyl alanine hydroxylase	Phenyl-ketone-uria (PKU)	Mental retardation, schizoid behaviour, light pigmentation, convulsions and eczema	Homozygous autosomal recessive	1:4000 – 1:60000 in different races and countries	(+)Ferric chloride test, Phenyl tyrosine raised in serum	Diet low in phenyl-alanine
(b) Histidine	Histidinase	Histidin-emia	Impaired speech and mental retardation	Heterozygous autosomal recessive	1:20000	Histidinase raised in serum (–) Ferric chloride test.	Diet low in histidine
(c) Methionine	Cystathionine β-synthetase Methylene-tetra hydrofolate reductase	Homo-cystinuria	Ectopic lens, Marfan-like features, coronary artery disease and mental retardation	Homozygous autosomal recessive	1:15000 – 1:30000	Raised serum methionine	Diet low in methio-nine
(d) Tyrosine	Homogentisi-case	Alkapton-uria	Black urine, black cartilage, blue ears, nose, cheeks, sclera arthritis, CVS disease and ochronosis	Homozygous autosomal recessive	1:100,000 – 1:200,000	Raised serum homogentisic acid and urine will show (+) Benedict and Fehling tests	High doses of ascorbic acid

Contd...

Table 8.1: Inborn errors of metabolism (*Contd...*)

S. No.	Enzyme (Protein)	Disorder	Clinical manifestation	Mode of inheritance	Incidence	Diagnosis	Treatment
(e) Tyrosine	Tyrosinase	Albinism two types Tyrosine(–) Tyrosine(+)	Fair skin, ocular problems, nystagmus, refractive errors, photophobia	Autosomal recessive and dominant and sex-linked non-allelic mutant genes in (–) Heterogenous in (+) cases		Appearance of painful burn of skin on being exposed to sunlight	Tyrosinase
2. Defects in Transportation of Aminoacids							
(a) Cystine	Not known probably cystein, lysine, arginine and ornithine can not be transported across the cell membrane	Cystinuria	Three types (I, II, and III) all with progressive renal colic and GIT obstruction	Type I autosomal recessive II and III incompletely autosomal recessive heterozygous	Rare	Raised urinary cystine with stones in kidney	Intake of plenty of fluid and pencillamine
(b) Cystine	Cystine reductase ISO-enzyme	Cystinosis	Three types, deposition of cystinosis crystals in reticulo-endothelial system, kidney and eyes, growth retardation, rickets, renal failure. Death in first decade by electrolyte imbalance.	Autosomal recessive heterozygous, homozygous for a mutant autosomal gene.		Raised cystine	Intake of plenty of fluids and penicillamine

Contd...

Table 8.1: Inborn errors of metabolism (*Contd...*)

S. No.	Enzyme (Protein)	Disorder	Clinical manifestation	Mode of inheritance	Incidence	Diagnosis	Treatment
3. *Defect in Metabolism of Carbohydrate*							
(a) Galactose and its variants	Glactose-I-phosphate uridyl transferase absent or inactive	Galacto-saemia	Child shows Hepatospleno-megaly, cataract, mental retardation, hypoglycaemia, low birth rated	Homozygous autosomal gene	1:16000	For absence of enzyme transferase in serum	Withdraw all sources of galactose
(b) Glucuronic acid (L-xylulose)	Reductase absent	Pentosuria	A-benign condition associated with emotional distur-bances, misdiag-nosed as diabetes mellitus, growth retardation, hepatomegaly.	Heterozygous autosomal recessive	1:40,000	L-xylulose accu-mulates in blood and excreted in urine about 1–4 gm per day reduction of Be-nedicts solution and similar reagents	Withdraw sources of glucuronic acid
(c) Glycogen storage di-sease, Cori type I-VI (Cori type 1, II, III, and V collectively) (von Gierke's disease)	In I, II, III Glu-cose-6-phos-phatase dehy drogenase enzyme and hepatic phos-phorylase in IV called as phosphorylase in V. Acid glucosidase in VI. Amyl-	Glycogenosis (Cori type-I) Forbes' disease (Cori-type-II), Her's disease (Cori type-III), muscle phosphorylase disease (Cori type-IV), Pompe's disease (Cori	McArdle's	X-linked (Cori type-I rest all auto-somal recessive but each as separate Mendelian character)	Not known commonest in Her's disease (Cori-III)	Depending upon the deficiency of enzyme, it varies, low blood glucose levels common to all	It varies in various types by dietary control

Contd...

Table 8.1: Inborn errors of metabolism (Contd...)

S. No.	Enzyme (Protein)	Disorder	Clinical manifestation	Mode of inheritance	Incidence	Diagnosis	Treatment
	pectinase, Glucogen synthetase deficiency	type-V) Andersons disease (Cori type-VI)		:			
	Over production of phosphoribosylamine leading to defective purine metabolism	Gout	Age of onset varies in males and females with average of 39-54 yr respectively. Acute attacks of inflammed swollen painful joint. Chronic gout shows granulomas and collection of sodium urate crystals in small joints of digits deforming hand and feet, chorea athetosis.	Sex-linked recessive males affected	Not known	Raised uric acid in blood (9.2–11 mg per 100 ml)	Probenecid which brings about reduction in blood uric acid
	Hypoxanthine guanine phosphoribosyltransferase	Gout	Age of onset children from 4–6 months, choreoathetoid movements starts after 6 months leading to spasticity, opisthotonus seizures.	Sex-linked recessive males-homozygous and females heterozygous	Not known	Raised uric acid in blood 8–15 mg/ 100 ml	Probenecid
4.	*Defects of Purine and Pyrimidine Metabolism*						

Contd...

Table 8.1: Inborn errors of metabolism (Contd...)

S. No.	Enzyme (Protein)	Disorder	Clinical manifestation	Mode of inheritance	Incidence	Diagnosis	Treatment
5. Lipid Metabolism (Lipidosis)	i. Glucocere-brosides a. Adult type b. Infantile c. Juvenile neurological form	Gaucher's disease, three types of normo-blastic ana-emia, neuro-logical prob-lem, throm-bocytopenia fragile bones leading to fractures, intercurrent infections, abnormal EEG, mental retardation, etc.	Age of onset: from 1 year to late in life, hepatosplenic	Autosomal recessive	Not known	Foam cells in bone, marrow	Not known
	ii. Hexosami-nidase A	Tay-Sachs disease or GM gangli-osidosis, or infantile amaurotic familial idiocy	Age of onset: 2–6 months or later, listless and hypo-tonic infant hy-peracusis with increasing eye changes in the form of degener-ated macule cerebral degen-eration, death by 5–8 yrs.	Autosomal recessive homozy-gous	One in 4000–6000 live births in Jews in USA, one in 3000–5000 live births in non-Jews in USA sligh-tly higher in Britain and Scandinavia	Reduce enzymes by assay of enzymes	Not known

Contd...

Table 8.1: Inborn errors of metabolism (*Contd...*)

S. No.	Enzyme (Protein)	Disorder	Clinical manifestation	Mode of inheritance	Incidence	Diagnosis	Treatment
	iii. Sphingo-myelinase sulfatase-A α galactosi-dase	Niemann Pick disease, sulphatide lipidosis, Fabry's disea-ses essential terolaemia (type II, etc.)	Hepatospleno-megaly, severe CNS damage Red spot on macula in ischaemic heart disease	Autosomal recessive Autosomal dominant hypercholes-terolaemia	40% in Jews	Reduce enzymes by assay of enzy-mes	Daily intra-venous in-fusions of 10,0,000,00 units of sulphatase B from ox brain Diet low in saturated fatty acids Infusion of plasma
6.	Mucopoly-saccharides (Mucopoly-sacchari-dosis)	Abnormal intracellular accumulation of mucopoly-saccharides	i. Hurler's syndrome Type I ii. Hunter's (Type II) iii. Sanfilippo syndrome iv. Morquio-Brailsford syndrome v. Scheie syndrome (type V) vi. Maroteaux-Lamy syndrome vii. Fucosidosis	Gargoyle facies, mental retardation, Hepatospleno megely, hearing defects, corneal clouding, CVS. problems, dwarfism and skeletal changes.	Autosomal recessive sex-linked (Type II) rest; all autosomal recessive		Excessive mucopoly saccharides diagnosed by culture of fibro-blasts from skin biopsy and WBC show metachromatic granules of acid mucopolysac-charides with toluidine blue staining	

Contd...

Table 8.1: Inborn errors of metabolism (*Contd...*)

S.No.	Disorder	Enzyme (Protein)	Clinical manifestation	Mode of inheritance	Incidence	Diagnosis	Treatment
7. *Minerals*	Wilson's disease (hepato-lenticular degeneration)	Copper	Age of onset: early childhood to sixth decade cirrhosis Kayser-Fleischer ring in cornea, neurological problem, jaundice prolonged renal osteoporosis, and osteomalacia	Autosomal recessive Heterozygous	Not known	Decreased serum ceruloplasmin and serum copper in some cases	BAL injection or oral penicillamine lead into decopperings liver transplant
	Haemochromatosis, haemoglobinopathies (it will be dealt as a separate entity under blood group chapter)	Iron	Age of onset: 20–35 yrs, sex—males generalised pigmentation, hepatomegaly, diabetes mellitus and endocrine disorders.	Familial	Not known	Raised serum iron	Phlebotomy to deplete body iron store or orally phosphate with food
8. *Defect of Membrane Transport (studied in three types of cells only in human being renal tubular epithelium, jejunal mucosas, erythrocytes)*	i. Renal glycosuria	Transport of glucose from renal tubules defective	Age of onset: childhood benign condition with excretion of glucose in urine leading to very low plasma concentration, kidneys are normal	Autosomal dominant	Not known	Abnormally low and flat glucose tolerance curve due to low absorption glucose from gut kidney	

Contd...

Table 8.1: Inborn errors of metabolism (*Contd...*)

S.No.	Enzyme (Protein)	Disorder	Clinical manifestation	Mode of inheritance	Incidence	Diagnosis	Treatment
		ii. Glucose-galactose malabsorption.	Age of onset within first week of life, severe diarrhoea stool being watery frothy and acid, dehydration leading to death (the symptom resemble those of alactasia)	Autosomal recessive	Not known	Low renal threshold for glucose differentiated from alactasia the stool contain glucose instead of lactose	Limited dietary carbohydrates except fructose
9.	Defective Absorption of Lysine, Arginine and Ornithine.	i. Cystinuria	Age of onset: 1–6 yr, kidney stones of cystine affected person are of small stature	Homozygous mutant autosomal gene	1–2500	Jejunal mucosae appear like renal tubular epithelium excretion of cystine, lycine and arginine increases in urine	Penicillamine therapy reduction of protein intake
		ii. Hartnup disease, phosphaturia or hypophosphataemic rickets Phosphoglucosaminoaciduria	Dermatitis, photosensitive, cerebellar ataxia, attacks of hallucination, delirium and fainting	Autosomal recessive, heterozygous	Not known	Low serum concentration of amino acid with excess in urine	Nicotinamide 15–65 mg/day throughout life

B. BLOOD GROUPS

The blood groups form an important part of human biochemical genetics but it is not possible to give a full account of all the presently known blood group systems. The understanding of underlying genetic principles forms an essential part of clinical diagnosis and management of affected individuals with defective and abnormal blood groups. The governing genetic principles are multiple allelism, codominance, polymorphism, linkage and immune reactions.

Transfusion of blood from one person to another was tried as early as 18th century in France and England, but the underlying basis of incompatibility in some cases was understood only in 1900 when Landsteiner classified all persons in universe to be belonging to an ABO blood group system, having four blood groups: A, B, AB, and O as given in the following table.

Genotype	Blood group
$i^0 i^0$	O
$I^A I^A$ or $I^A i^0$	A
$I^B I^B$ or $I^B i^0$	B
$I^A I^B$	AB

The concept of antigen and antibody was established at a later stage. At present there are at least more than one dozen blood group systems each controlled by an independent locus and at each locus there are multiple alleles. The various systems in use in order of frequency are described briefly.

ABO System

In this system only two types of surface antigens were recognised on the surface of red cells synthesized by three alleles—A, B and O present on chromosome 9. The person having the antigen A on red cell but antibody-B in serum belongs to blood group A, and reverse of this to group B, while when both A and B antigens with no antibodies in serum are present the blood group is AB and when no antigen with both A and B antibodies in serum are present the blood group is O. Thus the concept of persons with blood group O to be universal

Table 8.2: Agglutination reaction between donor's and recipient's blood

Blood group of donor	Blood group of recipient (agglutination reaction)			
	A	B	O	AB (Universal recipient)
A	(−)	(+)	(+)	(−)
B	(+)	(−)	(+)	(−)
AB (+)	(+)	(+)	(−)	(−)
O (Universal) donor	(−)	(−)	(−)	(−)

Blood group	Antigen	Antibody
A	A	B
B	B	A
AB	AB	Nil
O	Nil	AB

+ Clumping of red cell of recipient
− No clumping of red cells

Table 8.3: Possible blood group of children from parents of various blood groups of the ABO system

Blood group of parents M F	Possible blood group of children
O × O	O
O × A	O, A
O × B	O, B
O × AB	A, B
A × A	A, O
A × B	O, A, B, AB
A × AB	A, B, AB
B × B	B, O
B × AB	A, B, AB
AB × AB	A, B, AB

M = Mother, F = Father

donors and group AB to be universal recipient was formed as shown in Table 8.2 by the agglutination reaction between the donor's and recipient's blood during blood transfusion, as seen by clumping or no clumping of donor's red cells with the type of antibody present in the recipient's serum. The antibodies of donor's serum get so much diluted that they can not cause agglutination reaction of host red cells.

The genotype which produce these four blood groups is neither due to a dominant nor recessive gene but an intermediate gene, meaning thereby neither of the gene of these groups is dominant over the other and during inheritance can express itself in homo- as well as heterozygous forms.

Subtypes of ABO System

A number of subtypes of ABO blood group system are recognised on the basis of quantitative differences in their antigenicity (Table 8.3). These differences can be explained by knowing the steps involved in the formation of antigens as given below. The antigens A and B are formed by a precursor substance, which in turn is specifically synthesized by DNA as a specific enzyme protein for assembling the carbohydrate unit to produce specific blood group. The precursor substance is acted on by H-gene to produce H substance, which is further acted on by A or B gene to form the antigens for the blood groups A and B. If the genes A and B do not act on H substance it remains unchanged so no antigens for blood group O. If H gene does not act on precursor substance, no H substances is produced and we have the Bombay phenomenon described below. The steps are shown as follows.

Later on, it was found that gene A occurs at least in three all allelic from A1, A2, A3. This has also been shown that genes for A and B antigens are codominant while the gene for H antigen

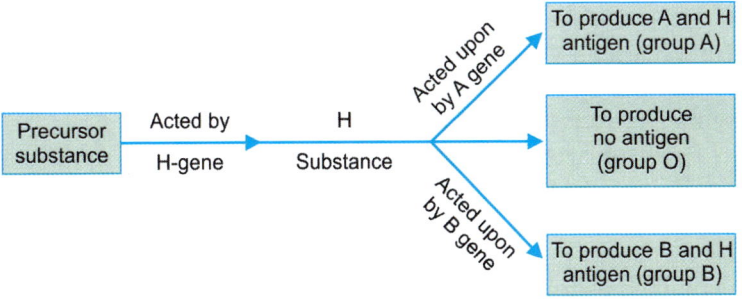

in blood group O is recessive. Similarly, the subgroup of A gene under the multiple alleles show an inter–relationship in the form of being dominant over each other as:

$A_1, A_2, A_3 = B > O$ on chromosome 9

Thus, this series of multiple alleles produce 8 phenotypes $A_1, A_2, A_3, B, A_1B, A_2B, A_3B$, and O with 15 genotypes, $A_1 A_1$; $A_1 A_2$; $A_1 A_3$; $A_1O, A_2A_2, A_2A_3, A_2O, A_3A_3, A_3O, A_1B, A_2B, A_3B$, BB, BO, and OO.

Bombay Phenotypes

Individual homozygous for inactive or amorph gene h are not able to form the A and B antigens, although the A and B genes are present. Antibody H is naturally found in such individuals (genotype hh). So the red cells of such individuals cannot be agglutinated by serum containing all the three types of antibodies A, B and H leading to confusion in judging the blood group. This type of individuals are very rare, and 1st case was reported in Bombay in 1952 and thus the named Bombay phenotype.

Rh Blood Group System

This second system discovered by Landsteiner and Weiner in 1940 by injecting immunised serum from Rhesus monkey in human blood (Table 8.4). The agglutination was evoked in 85% to 91% and the individuals were labelled as Rh +ve while the rest 9% to 15% with no agglutination were designated as Rh –ve. The exact genetic interpretation of Rh locus present on chromosome is not clear. According to Fischer and Race this blood group is determined by a series of closely linked genes C D E with allelic forms c d e giving eight possible combinations—Cde, cdE, cDe, CDe, cde, CDE, CdE and CdE. No naturally occuring antibodies are known for Rh antigen while Weiner designated the alleles as R and r.

Erythroblastosis foetalis: A haemolytic disease of newborn, (HDN) due to Rh incompatibility is characterised by jaundice and anaemia from 3rd day after birth with circulating erythroblasts in blood. The genetics of above condition can be explained as follows:

Table 8.4: Two notations used in Rh systems

Fisher and Race	Weiner
CDe	R_1
cde	r_2
cDE	R_0
CDe	R_1
Cde	r_1
cdE	r_4
CdE	r_1
CDE	r_2

When an Rh –ve woman carries an Rh –ve foetus and a break occurs in the barrier of placenta, separating maternal and foetal blood, the Rh antigen from the foetus finds its way into the maternal blood stream to stimulate the production of an antibody. This antibody does not react with the red cells of Rh –ve mother since there is no antigen, but the antibody finds its way through placenta to rh +ve foetus, where immunological reaction takes place between the antibody and the red cells of the foetus leading to haemolysis. Most of these haemolytic disease of newborn (HDN) are due to anti-Rh (anti-d) antibody. Few cases milder in form and thus difficult to diagnose are due to anti-A and rarely it can also be due to other blood group, antibodies like anti-K or anti-Fy^a. Antibodies like anti- Le^a and Le^b are found in serum of pregnant women but these are immunoglobulins which can not cross the barrier of placenta.

Rh Null Blood Group and D/D Genotype

In Australian aborigins, a very rare phenotype Bombay phenotype of ABO system was seen. There was no Rh antigen in these individuals as they do not have a precursor needed as a substrate for formation of antigens of rh system. They are homozygous for a rare X_r^0 whose allele X_r is responsible for synthesis of a precursor for both Rh and LW antigens. Similarly another rare Rh blood type when C and E series are missing and only D is present. This is deletion of C and E loci. However, the genotype is more likely to be due to a suppressor gene X^0.

Prophylaxis against Rh Immunisation

Rh sensitization usually occurs at the time of delivery or abortion, immunizing the mother by giving Rh_0 GAM, an anti-D antibody preparation before delivery or at the time of abortion, the sensitization of foetal cells can be almost completely prevented.

MNS Blood Goup System

In 1927, Landsteiner and Levine discovered the MN blood group after injecting rabbits with human red cells and used the resulting immune serum to distinguish other red cell samples. After about 20 years, i.e. in 1947 another antibody associated or related to M and N allele was discovered so that Ms Ns Ns combinations can occur (Table 8.5). The MNS antigens do not stimulate the antibodies in man and during blood transfusion, there will be no problem. There is no incompatibility between foetus and mother even. However, because of its relative frequency and codominance, the MNS system is the most useful blood group system medicolegally in disputed paternity or identity of individuals. The alleles M and N are found on chromosome 4 in homo- as well heterozygous forms.

At least fifteen well-defined red cell blood group systems of wide distribution in racial groups have been described, these are P Lutheran, Kell, Lewis, Duffy, Kidd, Diego and Yt, Xg, I and Dombrock, etc.

There are many other blood groups inherited by simple mendelian principles. The terminologies used in all these various blood groups are given in Table 8.6. In addition, a number of others, like August, Colton, Gerbich, Gregory, Lan and Vel, antigens have been described. The less frequent

Table 8.5: Combinations of blood group MN system for offsprings

			Mother		Phenotype	
		M	M	N		M
		M	M	M, MN		MN
Father	MN	MMN	M, MN, N	MN, N		
Phenotype	N	MN	MN, N	N		

antigens are named as private antigens while more frequent ones are called as public antigens. All these blood groups are of minor importance as regards the blood transfusion is concerned as compared to ABO system in general, and Rh system during pregnancy, and MNS system for disputed paternity in medicolegal cases. Similarly other blood groups are of significance in determination of zygosity twin studies, illegitimate children. X-blood group studies have added to the knowledge of sex chromosomal abnormalities and as regards the X-chromosome of maternal or paternal in origin. The phenomenon like monozygote heterokaryote, dispermy mosaicism producing chimeras although rare have been described in human beings by these studies. In addition, chromosomal mapping has also been developed by using the blood groups as marker genes and linkage studies of autosomes.

Blood Group Chimeras

A rare condition due to dizygotic twins or dispermic chimeras show two different types of blood cells by sharing their circulation during prenatal life. The exchange of blood cells takes place during foetal life before the development of immune system and thus no antibodies are formed against them and the cells remain dormant in bonemarrow of germ cells and exchanged during early developmental stage, otherwise the blood group of host is inherited.

Role of Blood Groups in Human Genetics

i. The blood group studies and their inheritance by simple Mendelian principle led to the understanding of genetics of normal traits.

ii. Defining the recessiveness and dominance of an allele, e.g. in K system of blood group, allele K was said to be dominant to the allele K once anti-K was discovered and allele K, its status was changed to codominant from recessive. Similarly, in ABO system presence of a suppressor gene suppressing the ABO allele was demonstrated in Bombay phenomenon.

Table 8.6: The features of other known blood groups

S. No.	Blood group	Notations (phenotype)	Used genotype	Discovery (year)	Remains
1.	P	P_1	$P_1/P_2P^1/p^1$	Landsteiner and Levin 1927	P^1 is dominant to P^2, while P and P^k are rare nondominant both like Bombay type. Frequency in Caucasians of P_1, P_2 is 79% and 21%.
2.	Lutheran	Lu^{a+b-} Lu^{a+b+} Lu^{a+b-} Lu^{a-b-}	Lu^a/Lu^b Lu^a/Lu^{ab} Lu_b/Lu^b Silent Lu gene	Callender et al. (1946) and Lutheran (1954)	A dominant suppressor gene, affects in the expression of all genes at Lu locus it has been the 1st gene, e.g. autosomal linkage of man, locus for myotonic dystrophy is also linked to Lu and sec loci
3.	Kell	K+ k	Kk, K_p^a, K_p^b	Coombs et al	J_3^a and J_3^b are never kk alin (1946 notations for antibodies), haemolytic disease of newborn (HDN) occasionally caused by foetomaternal interaction on Kk system.
4.	Lewis	Le^{a+b-} Le^{a+b+} Le^{a-b+} Le^{a+b+}	Le^{a+}, Le^{b+} silent rare, observed in adults	Maurant (1946)	Do not secret ABH. Always secretes ABH substance
5.	Duffy	Fy^{a+b-} Fy^{a-b+} Fy^{a-b-}	Fy^{a+} Fy^{b+} Fy^0	Contbush et al (1950)	1st locus to be closely linked to 'uncoiler' locus and assigned to chromosome 1, homozygous in 85% of Newyork blacks, having least susceptibility to malaria vivax parasite
6.	Kidd	Jk^{a+b+} Jk^{a-b+} Jk^{a-b-}	Jk^{a+} Jk^{b+} inhibitory or other gene	Allen et al (1951)	95% in West Africa, 93% in Negro (American), 77% in Europeans and 50% in others Anti-Jk^a is the cause of HDN and transfusion reactions

Contd...

Table 8.6: The features of other known blood groups (*Contd...*)

S. No.	Blood group	Notations phenotype	Used genotype	Discovery of year	Remains
7.	Digego	Di^{a+} Di^{a+} Di^{b+}	Di^a/Di^a Di^a/Di Di/Di	Layrisse *et al.* (1955)	Found in HDN. Specific marker for Mongolians Antigens are Anti diand di and Anti Di^b.
8.	I	I i	II, Ii ii	Weiner *et al.* (1956)	It is a 'cold antibody', i.e. active only at 4° temp. antigen differ from other blood groups in that some amount of antigen is present in all individual so and it increases from birth to reach adult levels by 18 months. The levels of antigen simultaneously fall, thus i antigen appears to be recessively inherited. Natural Anti-I does not cross the placenta. Anti-I has been found in cases of reticulosis and infectious mononucleosis.
9.	Xg	Xg^{a+} Xg^{a-}	Xg^a/Xg^a Xg^a/Y Xg/Xg, Xg/Y, (F) (M)	Weiner *et al.* 1956	It is X-linked dominantly inherited. The locus Xg has been of some use in mapping of chromosome X, but it appears not to take part in inactivation of X-chromosome. Icthiosis and ocular albinism are linked with Xg locus. It is also a marker gene and helps in population genetics to find the % age of X-linked genes.
10.	Yt or Y + (Cart fright)	Yt^{a+b-} Yt^{a+b+} Yt^{a+b+}	Yt^a/Yt^a Yt^a/Yt^b Yt^{a-b+}	Eaton *et al.* (1956)	98% are Yt^{a+}
11.	Dom-brock	Do^{a+b+} Do^{a+b+}	Do^a/Do^a Do^b/Do^b	Swanson *et al.* 1965	64% of northern Euro-peans are Do^{a+}

iii. Another branch of genetics, i.e. population genetics, developed by studying the distribution of various blood groups in different parts of world.

iv. In autosomal linkage studies, blood groups have been used as marker genes but recently other marker genes have also been found.

v. In modern surgery, safe blood transfusion is solely dependent on the understanding of blood group serology and genetics.

vi. Rh blood group system has led to the discovery of HDN and multiple allelism.

vii. The application of blood group serology in some important medicolegal cases like disputed parentage, and identification of blood stains in some criminal cases has served a useful purpose.

viii. The twin studies with its many genetic uses has been dependent on the underlying basis for blood group system.

Marker Genes and Disease Risks

It has been seen that the individuals with blood group A are having higher risk of getting pancreatic cancer, pernicious anaemia, salivary gland tumour and some tumours of ovaries. Blood group O individuals having risk of gastric and duodenal ulcers; individuals who are PTC tasters show raised risks of some thyroid diseases and one kind of glaucoma. These studies have led to the concept of marker genes, i.e. genes helping to identify the traits seen in an individual, family, and in generation.

Gene markers can be present on cells as well as serum, and are useful in medicolegal cases, population genetics and mapping of a chromosome.

The trait governed by a marker gene has to be highly polymorphic, has many codominant genes. Their mode of inheritance is simple and occurs in different frequencies in different population and the phenotype can be readily classified.

Classification of Genetic Markers

i. *DNA Markers*

Minor variations in DNA sequences can be picked up by restriction Endonucleases—named as Restriction Fragment Length Polymorphism (RFLP) and these variations form important markers.

ii. *Blood Group Markers*

According to an ICMR bulletin (1984), about 800 data sets are available under socioreligious and linguistic basis for various blood groups. In India, in general there is higher incidence of group B then group A, the people living near the borders of Bhutan, Nepal and Tibet have higher frequency of gene A and thus more frequency of Mongoloid features. In Indian population there is regional variation in frequency of ABO blood groups, i.e. Brahmins show different states indicating that they are not of same genetic composition. Similarly, the muslims and the tribals in different regions are heterogenous with respect to gene frequency of ABO blood groups. The regional variation in gene frequency seems to be greater than the variation between the castes or religious groups in the region.

ABO and disease association: It means two phenotypes are found together more often man expected, so that knowing one phenotype helps to predict the other, e.g. 40% of males with blood group 'O' are likely to get duodenal ulcers than males with blood group 'O' predisposes to duodenal ulcer.

Uses of blood group system as genetic markers:

a. Disputed paternity
b. Identification of newborns accidently changed in hospitals
c. Identification of the proportion of illegitimate children
d. Confirmation of pedigree information particularly when the condition under study is rare or when the other tests in carriers seem anomalous
e. Determination of zygosity twin, mono- or dizygosity

iii. *Genetic Markers in Serum*

Oliver and Smith in 1955 developed electophoretic techniques leading to discovery of many biochemical markers in serum of man, e.g. immunoglobulins, tranferrins and Xm serum system.

iv. *Human Lymphocyte Antigen System (HLA system)*

As marker is the most polymorphic system known in man. The antigen is present on chromosome 6. Chemically, the antigen is made up of heavy and light chains, and is useful for tissue typing. For organ transplantation in addition to tissue typing, tissue matching is an essential prerequisite. The HLA system is so polymorphic that an unrelated person can be rarely matched perfectly. The disease showing HLA associations include ankylosing spondylitis, juvenile diabetes, and autoimmune disease. Thus, HLA system forms an integral part of immunogenetics.

v. *Immunoglobulins as Markers*

These are inherited antigenic determinants in a immuno-globulin molecule. A γ-globulin molecule is composed of two identical light and two identical heavy chains held together by disulfide bonds. Immunoglobulins can be classified into five major classes: IgG, IgA, IgD, IgE and IgM.

vi. *Chromosomes as Markers*

The chromosomal variations seen during metaphase in a karyotype of an individual can be referred to as marker chromosome, e.g. philadelphia, fragile-X chromosome.

vii. *Hepatoglobulins as Markers*

These are globulins with the property of binding the haemoglobin and during crossing over, a slight shifting during pairing of homologous chromosomes leads to abnormal crossing and thus gene location. Hepatoglobulins are mutant allele by unequal crossing over known as α-globulins, concerned with the binding of haemoglobin from aged and broken red cells. The main differences arise due to variable α and β chains.

C. HAEMOGLOBINOPATHIES

In human beings, the disorders produced due to abnormal synthesis (Fig. 8.2) of the haemoglobin molecule can be classified into two main groups:

1. *Structural haemoglobinopathies:* When the protein subunits are structurally abnormal.
2. *Thalassaemias:* Where the rate of synthesis of subunits is unbalanced.

The normal haemoglobin molecule is a tetramer of four polypeptide chains: two α and two β chains (Fig. 8.3). Mutations giving rise to change in sequence of amino acids either by deletion or substitution leads to these haemoglobinopathies. The molecular weight of Hb molecule is 64500 daltons and in human beings there are atleast six different globin polypeptide chains coiled and folded in a complex manner and contains a heam group—a porphyrin ring with an iron atom at the centre that combines with oxygen. The α chain has 141 amino acids and β chain has 146 amino acids (Fig. 8.4). The sequence in both the chains is similar though not identical. The sequence of amino acids is termed primary structure, the helical coiling is the secondary structure, the folding complexity forming pocket for heme is the tertiary structure, and finally the four chains are associated to form a globular structure of Hb and thus its function depends on collective forces of four factors as follows:

i. A large a helical content (75%) of each chain.
ii. The firm binding of the heme group in its pocket.
iii. The internal sitting of the nonpolar amino acids determining the folding of the chain.
iv. The stability of the contacts holding the a and b chains together.

The genes for various Hbs are present on chromosomes 11 and 16 as shown in Fig. 8.2 both normal and abnormal with some having one locus and other having two loci for various chains to produce tetramers.

Types of Haemoglobin Seen Normally in Human Beings

Haemoglobin molecule in adult constituting about 98% of total Hb is denoted as HbA or (α-2 β-2 polypeptide chain).

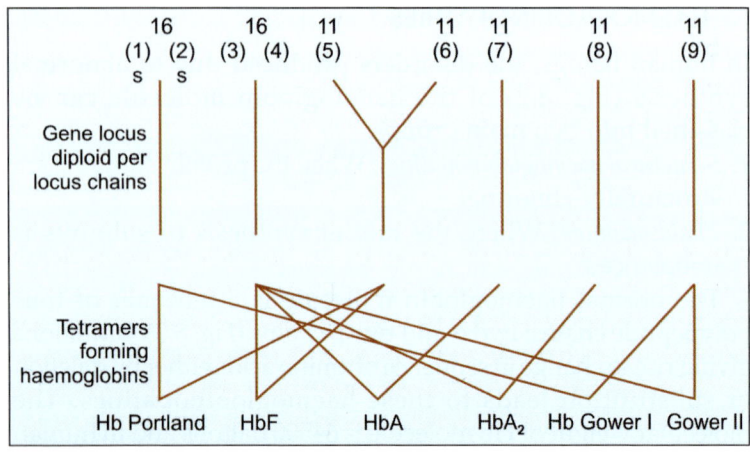

Fig. 8.2: Various normal and abnormal haemoglobin loci on various chromosomes

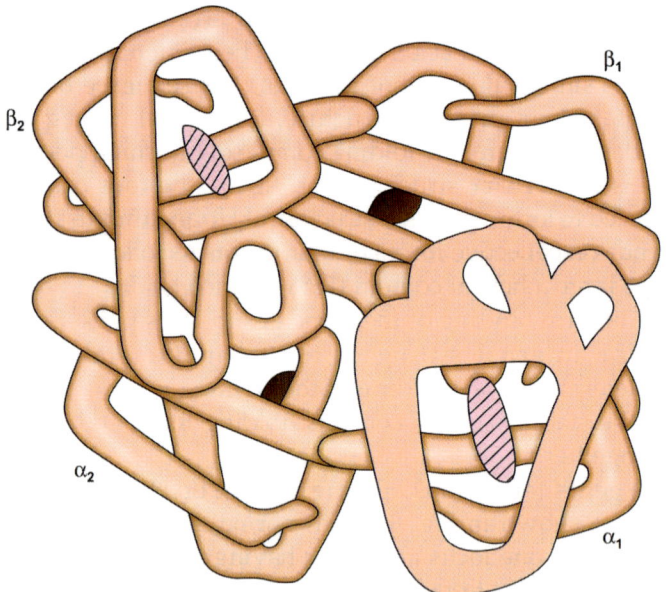

Fig. 8.3: Haemoglobin molecule

HbA$_2$ is the minor adult Hb (2%), has two α and two δ chains. During foetal life HbF is the major part constituting about 80%

of total Hb at the time of birth, which is rapidly replaced by HbA during the first few months of extrauterine life. HbF has two α and two γ chains, embryonic Hb appears transiently in very early stage of development and is no longer seen after 8 cm C.R. length. Embryonic Hb has three varieties—Gower I (σ-2, θ-2 chains), Gower II (α-2, θ-2 chains), and Portland (σ-2, γ-Z).

HbH and Barts are tetramers of β and γ chains respectively and are very poor in oxygen transport.

In haemoglobinopathies (Table 8.7), the abnormal function of Hb can be classified into:

1. Unstable Hbs
2. Hbs with increased oxygen affinity
3. Hbs with reduced oxygen affinity
4. Methaemoglobin

The mutations at primary structure of Hbs can ultimately lead to substitution at other three levels leading to a number of variants are haemoglobinopathies. These studies have also helped in chromosomal mapping and gene regulation.

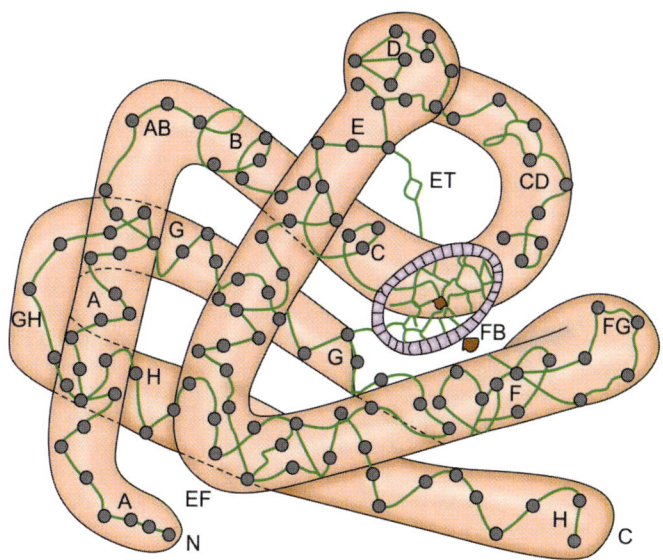

Fig. 8.4: β chain of HbH

The thalassaemias are the group of inherited anaemias characterised by a failure of haemoglobin polypeptide chains production in normal quantities. In normal adult, the polypeptide chain synthesis is so regulated that output of α- chains is equal to the combined output of β and δ chains. The latter synthesis proceeding at approximately 1/5th the rate of former. The rate of synthesis in turn depends on production of mRNA, unable to read ribosomes, the tRNA deficiency may lead to abnormality of amino acids being added to the polypeptide chain, etc. The first disorder of such nature discovered was called as Cooley's anaemia or thalassaemia major, or target cell anaemia, microcythaemia or mediterranean anaemia the other forms known are α thalassaemia, β thalassaemia, etc.

Hereditary persistance of foetal Hb is an entirely symptomless condition, and F-gene inheritance in high doses prevents the change from γ chain to β chain production after birth. Heterozygotes have 10–15% of HbF and low HbA level: homozygotes have HbF only. The practical importance of this condition lies in misdiagnosing as thalassaemia, if the only Hb levels are considered.

D. IMMUNOGENETICS

The underlying basis of immunity is the capacity of an individual to recognise what is *self* and what is *non-self*. This

Table 8.7: Various types of Hbs in human beings

Name	Formula	Percentage	Remarks
Adult			
HbA	$\alpha_2\mu_2$	98%	
HbA$_2$	$\alpha_2\beta_2$	2%	Replaces foetal Hb
Foetal			
HbF	$\alpha_2\gamma_2$ 136 Gly	80%	Replaced by adult Hb
	$\alpha_2\beta_2$ 136 ale	20%	
Embryonic			
Hb Gower II	$\alpha_2\varepsilon_2$	not known	Replaced by Foetal Hb
Hb Gower I	$\chi_2\varepsilon_2$	not known	
Portland	$\chi_2\gamma_2$	not known	

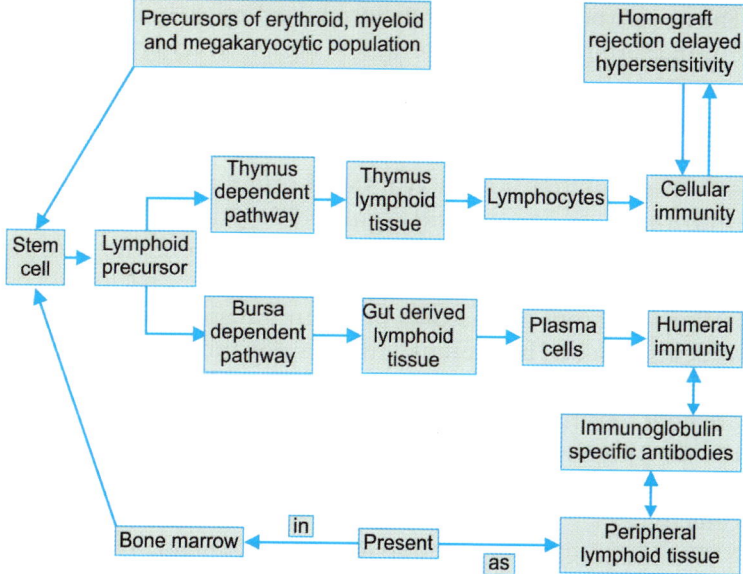

Fig. 8.5: Simplified outline of the pathways of differentiation of cells involved in the immune response

capacity is vital for survival. When any bacteria or virus or cancer cell invades the body, the body recognises these invaders as *non-self* and tries to destroy them before any damage to body is done. In human beings, the appearance of lymphoid tissue by about 12 weeks of intrauterine life is considered to be the beginning of immune defence capability. Basically there are two types of systems for a stem cell (Fig. 8.5):

i. The Bursa system or "B-cells" responsible for the production of circulating antibody–an immunoglobulin, to combat the bacterial and viral infection toxins and some particulate matter as antigens.

ii. The thymus system or "T-cells" responsible for cellular immunity plays a major role in transplantation and represents a factor in the natural defense mechanism against bacterial, viral, fungal and protozoal and probably cancer cells.

In Bursa system, when a foreign body enters the body it is engulfed by the macrophage by a nonimmunological process.

The foreign body is either transformed or broken into fragments by macrophages. They are taken up by small lymphocytes converting them to lymphoblasts and then to plasma cells which are now called as B-cells.

The T-cells, on other hand, are known as 'memory cells' and live in circulation for 10 years and bring about the cellular immunity. It has recently gained importance in organ transplantation, in which the sequence of events for foreign cells will be same as seen by the invasion of a bacteria. The antigens present on the cells of organ transplant are detected as being non-self by the small thymus dependent lymphocytes after being processed by the macrophages. These lymphocytes are now sensitised and transrformed into lymphoblasts, which divide into new lymphocytes, each one sensitised to grafted cells of organ and bearing antibodies against the foreign organ cells.

The antibodies in cellular immunity remain fixed to the lymphocytes and initiate the rejection of non-self grafted cells by enlisting the aid of macrophages. The immune response may turn against some patients and induce damage, e.g. rheumatic fever and glomerulonephritis. The other extreme of body not responding to a foreign antigen by developing tolerance instead of immunity and accept the antigen as self. This occurs in immunologically immature or deficient individuals, e.g. in dizygotic twins who may exchange blood cells precursors in utero and thus become histocompatible. The concept of tolerance is particularly relevant to the organ transplantation.

The antibodies are manufactured by the plasma cells and they function on the basis of their physico-chemical properties. The genetic mechanism by which the body can produce the antibodies is still under intense investigations. The antibodies after being formed are released in circulation and are capable of combining specifically with the corresponding antigen.

These antibodies known as immunoglobulins, based on their physico-chemical properties, can be classified into five classes— IgG, IgM, IgA, IgD and IgE (Table 8.8).

The immunoglobulins represent about 20% of total serum proteins and 75% of these belong to IgG group, which takes part in reactions against a variety of bacteria, viruses, and toxins. Next 15% is IgA, secreted locally into saliva, intestinal juice, colostrum and respiratory secretions. IgM, about rest 10% is prominent in early immune responses. IgD and IgE forming about only a fraction of 1%, latter probably involves in allergic reactions or diseases and effect of IgD is still unclear, but some reports have associated it with antibodies against insulin, thyroid, milk proteins, penicillin and diphtheria toxoid. IgM is the predominant immunoglobin on the surface of B-cells. The persons are said to be immune to a certain infection which is manifested by the immunological memory given by B-cells. On antigenic stimulation *memory* is rapidly translated into the activity of antibody production. The memory cell immediately recognises the M substance of type of organism.

An IgG is structurally a heavy chain and nearly twice as long as the light chain (Fig. 8.6). Heavy chain is further divided into two equal parts by papain digestion. The C-terminal half, i.e. Fc fragment is constant while the N-terminal half Fd fragment is variable, being divided into again two halves. The half towards C-terminal being constant but the half towards N-terminal is variable. This variable part of heavy chain is spatially related to the variable half of light chain and these both

Table 8.8: Human immunoglobulins with some properties

Properties	Name of immunoglobulins				
	IgG	IgM	IgA	IgD	IgE
Molecular weight (kDa)	160,000	900,000	170,000-390,000	190,000	190,000
Plasma level (mg/100 ml)	900-1500	70-100	150-400	0.3-4.0	0.01-0.06
Name and formula of chains	Heavy chain	Meiu	Alfa	Delta	Epsilon
	γ	μ	α	δ	ϵ
	$\gamma_2\kappa_2$	$(\mu_2\kappa_2)_5$	$\alpha_2\kappa_2$	$\delta_2\kappa_2$	$\epsilon_2\kappa_2$
	or	or	or	or	or
	$\gamma_2\lambda_2$	$(\mu_2\gamma_2)$	$\alpha_2\lambda_2$	$\delta_2\lambda_2$	$\epsilon_2\lambda_2$
Transplacental passage	Yes	No	No	No	No
Serum Half-life (days)	26	5	6	3	2

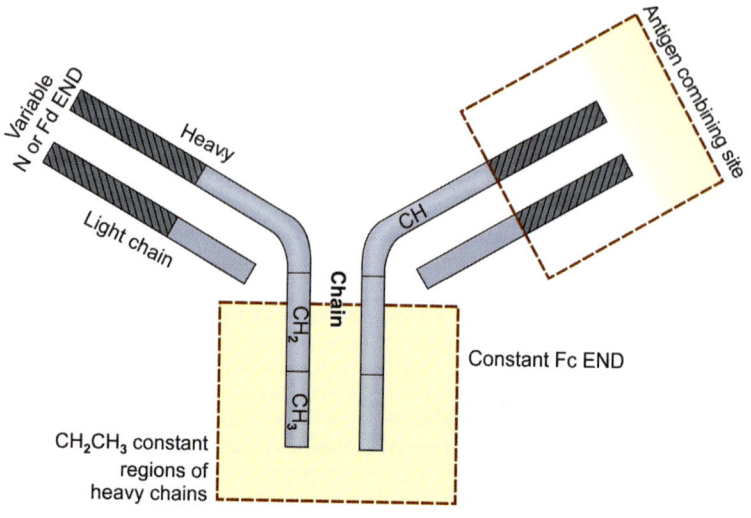

Fig. 8.6: Immunoglobulin molecule

contribute to the specific antigen-binding site of antibody molecule. Inherited variations in aminoacid sequence usually occur in k-light chain (INV type) and in y (Gm type) and A (Am types) heavy chains. These variations known as allotypes are serologically distinguishable. The loci for both heavy and light chains are autosomal and not closely linked except the heavy chains of IgG and IgA which are very closely linked.

None of the immunoglobulin allotypes is known to have any direct relationship with a particular disease. However, there are several clinical syndromes associated with the inherited traits primarily due to immunological deficiency states.

Some of the known syndromes are:

1. *Sex-linked agammaglobulinaemia of Burton:* Where all classes of immunoglobulins are deficient leading to mesenchymal diseases, rheumatoid arthiritis, scleroderma, dermatomyositis, and diffuse vasculitis.

2. *Ataxia telangiectasia:* The deficiency is mainly of IgA and IgE because of ataxia, occlocutaneous telangiectases, and impaired hypersensitivity response.

3. *Swiss type of alymphocytic agammaglobulimaemia:* Inherited as autosomal recessive with both cellular and humoral

immunological responses impaired and is thus more pernicious. Thymic hypoplasia and marked deficiency of lymphocytes is characteristic.

4. *Wiskott–Aldrich syndrome:* Inherited as X-linked recessive disorder characterised by eczema, thrombocytopenia and marked susceptibility to infection. The deficiency is of IgM due to reduced ability of lymphoid to process antigen for stimulation of IgM formation.

E. PHARMACOGENETICS

"What is food to one is bitter poison to other" as said by Lucretius. It is a known fact that individuals vary in their response to drugs. It should not be surprising since the whole sojourn of the drug, i.e. from its rate of absorption to reach the target organ and metabolism for excretion across the cell membranes is governed by genes and modified by environment (diet and other drugs, etc). Sometimes the response of an individual to a particular drug is so much away from normal response that it becomes life threatening. Such marked deviations in response show simple Mendalian inheritance leading the German geneticist Vogal in 1952 to name this branch of genetics as pharmacogenetics—a special form of inborn errors of metabolism. There are a number of conditions involving abnormal reactions to drugs which show simple Mendalian inheritance, shown in Table 8.9. There are certain diseases which may get precipitated by certain drugs (Hutington's chorea, porphyria, etc). It is likely that further genetic differences to drugs will be found thus allowing increasing accuracy in determining doses, choosing appropriate drugs and avoiding undesirable side reactions. The principles underlying pharmacogenetics may act as an aid to classify certain disorders.

Table 8.9: Some inherited conditions with altered response to some drugs

S. no.	Drug	Altered response	System involved	Trait or deficient enzyme seen
1.	H_2O_2	No response to peroxide	Tissues	Acatalasia
2.	Alcohol	Increased tolerance	Liver	Alcohol dehydrogenase
3.	Smoking other air pollutants	Emphysema	Lungs cirr-hosis liver	α-1-antitrypsin deficiency
4.	Chlopro-pamide	Flushing after alcohol ingestion	Vasomotor	Diabetes mellitus
5.	Dicumorol	Decreased response	Clotting	Dicumorol resistance
6.	Glucocorticoids	Increased ocular pressure	Eye	Glaucoma
7.	Anti-malarial, primaquin or Fava beans or others	Haemolysis	RBC	Glucose-6-phosphate dehydrogenase
8.	Chlorthiazide (diuretic)	Exacerbation of gout	Uric acid metabolism	Gout
9.	Sulfonamide, oxidants	Haemolysis	RBC	Unstable haemoglobins
10.	Levodopa	Tremors in "gene carriers"	Brain	Huntington's chorea
11.	Isoniazid	Polyneuritis	Liver	1-NH transacetylase
12.	Anesthetics	Riger	Sarcoplasmic reticulum	Malignant hyperthermia
13.	Nitrites	Methaemo-globinaemia	RBC	Methaemoglobin reductase
14.	Insulin, Adrenaline and others	Paralysis	Cell mem-brane	Periodic paralysis
15.	Barbiturates, sulfas and others	Acute attack	Liver	Some kinds of porphyria
16.	Succinyl-choline	Apnoea	Plasma liver	Pseudocholinesterase deficiency

EXERCISE

1. Enumerate the fields covered under biochemical genetics.
2. What do you understand by one gene one enzyme concept by Beadle Tatum?
3. Draw a flow chart to show the metabolic steps of phenylalanine metabolism. Highlight the levels of blocks which can occur at various steps to produce its effects.
4. Enumerate or classify inborn errors of metabolism.
5. Write short notes on:
   a. PKU
   b. Multiple allelism
   c. Polymorphism
   d. Codominance.
6. Fill in the blanks.
   a. Blood transfusion was tried as early as .... century in France and England but was understood only in .... century by discovery of .... blood group system.
   b. Rh locus is present on chromosome ....
   c. The haemolytic disease of the new born due to .... is characterised by .... and .... from 3rd day after birth is called ....
   d. Rh .... to mother is usually given during .... and .... trimesters of pregnancy/ abortion by giving .... antibody.
7. Match the following:

   i. Acatalasia   a. Transplacental passage
   ii. IgG   b. $\alpha_2\gamma_2$
   iii. Lymphocyte T   c. Chromosome 16 and 1
   iv. HbF   d. Adult Hb
   v. Abnormal Hb loci   e. H_2O_2
                                    f. Cellular immunity

9

Clinical Genetics

All diseases in human can be classified into following headings.

i. *Purely genetic in origin, e.g. inborn errors of metabolism*

ii. *Both genetic and environmental in origin, e.g. pyloric stenosis*

iii. *Purely environmental in origin, e.g. tuberculosis, etc.*

The understanding of first two types of diseases are gaining more importance because of the control of third type of diseases by improved health conditions and discovery of better and new drugs. Although, the first type of diseases are rarer and their mode of transmission is simple Mendalian but of high-risk recurrence and type two diseases are commoner and the mode of inheritance is multifactorial with low risk of recurrence.

Under this chapter, thus the branches like population genetics, dermatoglyphics, genetic counselling and experimental genetics are required to be dealt.

I. POPULATION GENETICS

It is the science dealing with the study of genes in a population as regards their distribution, behaviour and frequency with variations, etc. The changes seen in various genotypes are the basis for evolution. A geneticist experiments on insects, plants or animals to reach to a conclusion but a human geneticist is not able to do any direct laboratory observations because of the longer time period of one generation in human beings, i.e. about 25 years. However, it has been seen that people from different parts of world show an infinite range of genetic variability of different traits, and these can be observed instantaneously and the frequency calculated mathematically and statistically.

The definition of the term race in world population is a group of people more or less isolated geographically or culturally, sharing a common gene pool, statistically are somewhat different at some loci from others in the population. The analysis of genes in a population for a beginner pedigree analysis. Surprisingly, the most powerful tool for genetic analysis is an algebraic test of frequencies of genotypes and phenotypes in total number of loci present in human species, numbering about one lakh. All but a small number is common to all groups. A small number of alleles in skin colour in African, Oriental and European populations are obvious examples. These allelic differences represent a minute fraction of total loci. There is no case known in human beings when an important allele is present in one group and not in other.

Hardy-Weinberg Principle

There are numerous genes in human beings, some advantageous and other deleterious. From this pool of genes, an individual draws two genes for each locus at random. The probability or frequency of such genes in a population has been algebraically worked out by GH Hardy, a mathematician and W Weinberg, a physician independently in 1908.

There are three statements under the Hardy–Weinberg equilibrium, law or principle:

a. In a population in equilibrium, the frequency of a disease caused by a homozygous gene is the square of frequency of that gene, provided the frequency of gene is known in the population.

b. The frequency of a gene in a population in equilibrium will be the square root of the frequency of homozygotes for that gene.

c. The frequency of heterozygotes for two alleles is the frequency of one allele multiplied by frequency of other allele two times.

In algebraic terms this law states that in a population in equilibrium if a genetic locus has alleles D and d with frequencies p and q respectively, the frequencies of genotypes DD, Dd and dd will be p2 square, two pq, and q respectively.

Now there are factors altering the frequencies of genes and thus disturbing the Hardy–Weinberg rule and they are mutation, selection, blind balance between the two, genetic heterogeneity, heterozygote advantages, segregation ratio, advantage and genetic drift, etc. The rate of mutation producing a variation is very low (one per million) but natural selection will increase the frequency of advantageous genes and decrease that of deleterious ones. Similarly, in small populations the gene frequencies in one generation may not coincide with those in the next because of a random selection of a small number of gametes from the populations of gametes may just happen to result in a higher or lower percentage of allele than in the previous generation. This is basically statistical or chance phenomenon and is known as genetic drift.

The Hardy–Weinberg equilibrium is also disturbed with *random mating*. In practice, the required random mating if not normally fulfilled and there is a preferrential selection of a mate either by positive nonrandom mating or by a negative non random mating. Consanguineous mating is a special form of assortative mating where the Hardy–Weinberg equilibrium is disturbed by reducing the heterozygotes and thus increasing the proportion of homozygotes.

Factors altering the Hardy–Weinberg equilibrium:

a. *Mutation:* It brings about change in genetic constitution of an individual from one stable state to another state. This change can be beneficial during evolution, but mostly the change is harmful and can be compared to throwing a monkey wrench into a running machine which would hardly improve the function of machine.

b. *Selection and balance between selection and mutation:* The more harmful a mutation, the stronger is the selection against it and less frequent is the gene. Thus the frequency of any given allele reflects a balance between the rate at which alleles of this kind are being removed from population by selecting naturally, and the rate at which new ones are being created by mutation.

c. *Heterozygote advantage and genetic heterogeneity:* In dominant mutations, the mutant allele is so rare that homozygotes can be ignored and in recessive mutations, the mutant gene does not affect the fitness of heterozygote. This leads to increase in frequency of the recessive mutant gene. Genetic heterogeneity means the similar phenotypes produced by two genotypes.

Genetic drift: It is the fluctuation in gene frequency occurring usually in a small population. Gene flow is a gradual diffusion of genes from one population to another by migration.

Charles Darwin, the father of evolution, gave a statement of *survival of fittest* considering the relative ability of an organism to survive and transmit its gene to the next generation. It is determined by the number offsprings reaching the reproductive age and it is 100% if a person has atleast two such offsprings. The dominant genes which are always expressed than the recessive genes and are readily measured by obvious effects selectively.

MULTIPLE BIRTHS AND THEIR USES IN GENETICS

Man and other large mammals normally produce only one offspring at a time. Twins have always been a subject of interest yet it was only in 1875 that Galton pointed out their value in genetics while working on heredity and environment in *nature and nurture*. The monozygotic, dizygotic and mossaic twins acted to compare genetically similar or different or a combination of both. The incidence of twin births varies in different parts of world but overall incidence is 1: 80–90 with incidence of identical twins as 1:270. The incidence of monozygotic twins is surprisingly constant ranging from 3.5 to 4 per thousand deliveries in various populations, the cause of these identical twins is still not known. The variation in frequency of dizygotic twins is thought to be due to a number of factors like age, and race on different geographical regions. The familial tendency is seen in dizygotic twins only and not in monozygotic twins. When the twins are used to estimate heritability, the zygosity must be determined by examining the fetal membranes and physical similarity, dermatoglyphic patterns, genetic marker, skin grafts, etc.

Unusual twins are born due to a number of factors during the early developmental stages, e.g. blood group chimeras due to exchange of cells in dizygotic twins, in Siamese twins, where there is late separation of dividing cells into two different groups to produce twins, monozygotic twins born by super fecundation by two different fathers, and even monozygotic twins of different phenotypes are known to occur due to mitotic non-dysjunction during early stages of development with a loss of one sex chromosome giving rise to either one XY, another XO or one XX and another XO twin. Genetic predisposition of an infectious disease or allergy or cancer in twins has also been studied and found to be more in monozygotic twins.

Monozygotic twins are thus a rich source of genetic material for analysing the effects of environment on genes.

II. DERMATOGLYPHICS

It is the science which deals with the study of dermal ridge configuration on the digits, palms and soles. These patterns start developing as early as thirteenth week of intratuterine life in the form of mounds on the tips of digits, interdigital, thenar and hypothenar areas of hands and as regressed areas on the corresponding regions of soles. The pattern formation is complete by the ninteenth week of IUL. Walker was first to demonstrate the typical pattern in case of Down's syndrome. Since then a number of other syndromes has been extended the similar approach but some of them are invalid. Even if a specific syndrome may not be diagnosed still it seems to be a useful screening procedure specifically in Down's syndrome and abnormal pattern has some diagnostic value as a sign of disturbed prenatal growth, e.g. in cases of mental retardation whether the cause is perinatal or prenatal.

Terminology Used in Dermatoglyphic

a. *Finger tip pattern:* They are mainly of three to four types, classified by the number of *triradii* present, which is a point present at the confluence of ridges going in different direction like a fork (Fig. 9.1). A simple arch has no triradius while a tented arch has a central triradius. The loop has a single triradius and is called ulnar or radial depending on the side to which it opens. The whorl has two or more triradii and may be a double loop or more commonly a circular type of pattern. The ridge count in finger tips is done between the centre of pattern and the farthest triradius, thus arches have a zero count while the whorls have the highest count and the total ridge count (TRC) is the sum of the ridges on all the ten finger tips. Conventionally the digits are numbered from thumb to little finger. The frequency of any pattern varies in various tips of right or left side, e.g. the arches and loops, specially radial ones have the lowest frequency but when present occur commonly on digit tip 2, whorls occur most often on digits 4, 1 and 2 and females have more arches and few whorls than males. There are also racial differences (Figs 9.2 and 9.3).

b. *Palmar patterns:* Palm can be divided into thenar, hypothenar and four interdigital areas. Normally, a thiradius is present at the base of palm between the thenar and hypothenar areas, known as axial triradius (t) and the four digital triradii a, b, c, and d are near distal border of palm and the main lines of interdigital areas as shown in Fig. 9.2 which is the normal pattern most commonly seen. The angle ATD is either measured, or the distance of palmar triradius from the distal wrist crease to proximal crease at the base of third digit is measured. Zero to 14% height is called normal t, 15 to 39% is t', and more than 40% is t" at any age group while the ATD angle if less than 46° is V and if more than 63° is t' (Figs 9.2 and 9.3).

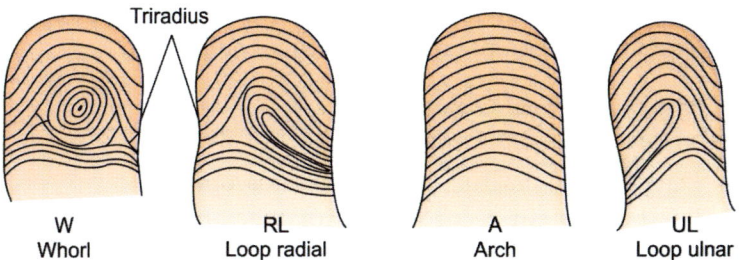

Triradius

| W | RL | A | UL |
| Whorl | Loop radial | Arch | Loop ulnar |

Fig. 9.1: Triradius and finger tips patterns

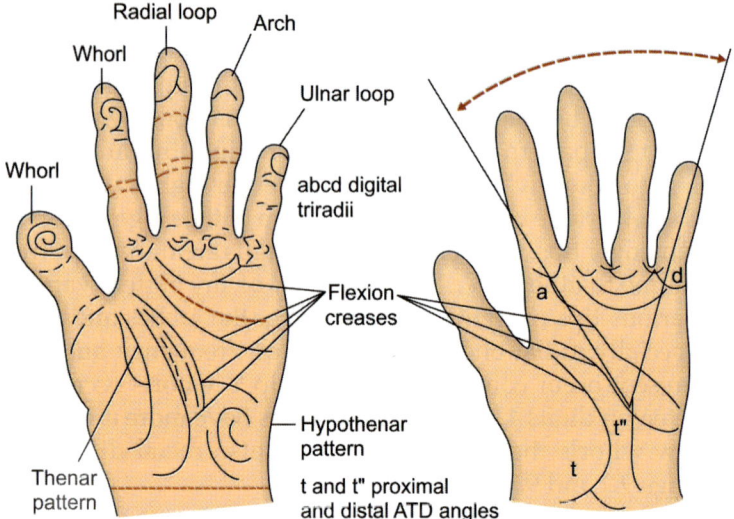

Fig. 9.2: Various dermal patterns in palm

Fig. 9.3: ATD angle > than 75° in Down's syndrome (normal 60°)

c. *Patterns on sole* (Fig. 9.4): The pattern observations are confined to hallucal areas, because of difficulties encountered for footprints. The most common pattern seen on hallux is the whorl, large distal loop and ridge count more than 21. Arch tibial is typically seen in Down's syndrome.

d. *Flexion creases:* These are dermatoglyphic patterns which are commonly included in analysis (Fig. 9.3). These are actually the dermal attachments to underlying structures and appear between 7th and 14th week of IUL. They are normally a distal and proximal transverse crease and a thenar crease. Figure 9.4 shows the typical dermal pattern in Down's syndrome, with simian crease on palm and arch tibial on hallux.

Methods Used for Obtaining the Dermatoglyphic Patterns

a. Directly by a magnifying glass of otoscope.

b. For permanent records and for measuring the various parameters, a number of techniques for printing are available with ink pads or inkless methods.

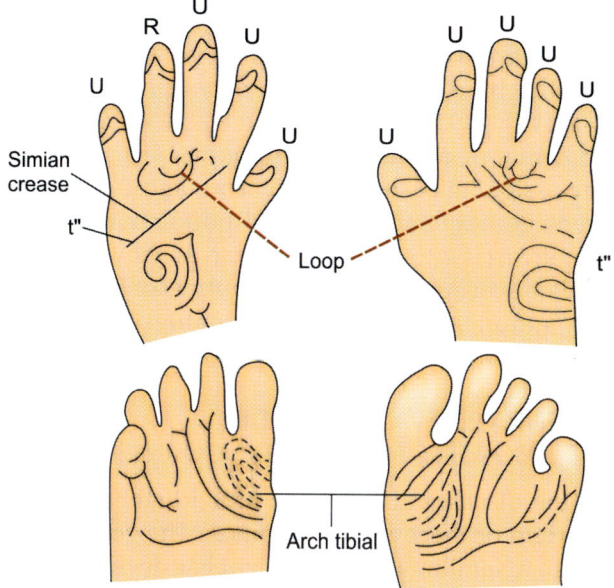

Fig. 9.4: Typical dermal pattern in Down's syndrome

Uses and Limitations of Dermatoglyphic Analysis

Similar dermatoglyphic patterns in monozygotic twins and unique finger prints of an individual suggest that the patterns are genetically determined as demonstrated by correlation of ridge count between various members of same family. Thus it is expected that the dermatoglyphic pattern will alter when a large number of genes are either missing or are in excess, and diagnostic value in some chromosomal syndromes when the patterns are consistent ones. The zygosity of twins can be diagnosed easily by several methods. The patterns on one digit although has no relation with pattern on other digit in the same individual, but there is a tendency for them to be alike, if they were independent of one another. [Neglecting these points and using too small a sample, failure to match control populations for race and sex and inappropriate use or non-use of statistical tests can lead to confusion as can be seen in cases of congenital heart disease, leukaemia and schizophrenia.]

Abnormal Dermatoglyphics

When evaluating a dermatoglyphic pattern without having any syndrome in mind, so that the severity of pattern as regards abnormality (Fig. 9.5) and whether the abnormality affects are developmental or not, a rough guide has been described by Perus by assigning each feature a score and the reciprocal of its percentage frequency in general population is multiplied by 10 to convert it into a whole number, as shown in Tables 9.1 and 9.2. For scoring method, distribution of normal control, with the summerised unusual dermatoglyphic pattern in various syndromes are shown in Tables 9.3 and 9.4.

ASSESSMENT AND EVALUATION OF GENETIC DISORDERS FOR GENETIC COUNSELLING

Most of the diseases affecting an individual can be either of genetic origin or there are other causes. The genetic disorders usually run in families unless a patient has developed a genetic disorder as the first proband case in the family tree. Hence, the suspected cases of genetic disorders have to be assessed carefully.

The following methods have to be taken into consideration for the assessment.

   i. **Family history:** After taking the routine history of the patient, which includes the personal, present and past, a

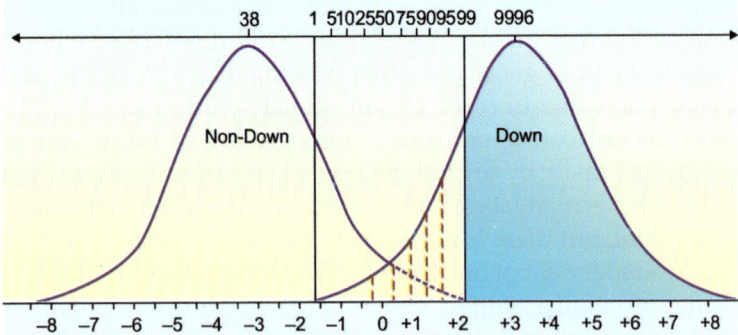

Fig. 9.5: A simple dermatoglyphic screening test for Down's syndrome

Table 9.1: Scoring method of quantifying the degree of abnormality in dermatoglyphic patterns

Area	Pattern	Score*
Digits	8–10 W	1
	7–10A	6
	4–6A	2
	RL on I (score once only)	25
	RL on III (score once only)	2
	RL on IV or V (score once only)	3
	10 UL	3
Hallucal	Tibial A or vestigial distal L	17
	A other than tibial L	17
	A other than tibial	1
	Tibial L	1
	Fibular L	4
	Distal L with fibular L under it	10
Palm	t bilateral	2
	t unilateral	1
	Thenar L, bi- or unilateral	2
	12 Pattern bi-or unilateral	6
	Thenar exit to A-line, bilateral	5
	Thenar exit to A-line, unilateral	2
	Absent, fused, misplaced triradius a, b or d	6
	Absent triradius	1
	Simian crease, bilateral	6
	Simian crease, unilateral	3
	Sydney line, bilateral	5
	Sydney line, unilateral	2

*The score is the reciprocal of the percentage frequency of the trait in the general population × 10.

detailed family history of the patient is taken for revealing whether any other member of family suffers from similar or any other genetic defect or disorder. In the obstetrical history of mother, exposure to X-rays or drugs during pregnancy or in the past history of patient to evaluate the environmental etiology for genetic mutation, can be taken.

ii. **Pedigree charting:** For family history recording, there are a number of ways accepted but at Department of Human

Table 9.2: Cumulative distribution of dermatoglyphic scores for normal controls

Score	% of control	% of control with this or lower score
<1	20	20
1–2	44	64
3–4	14	78
5–6	10	88
7–8	6	94
9–10	3	97
11	3	100

Genetics, University of Michigan Medical School, a method has been adapted, accepted internationally by using symbols (*see* Fig. 7.1), so that the family history information can be read quickly without any loss of clarity and accuracy. Variations of symbols or some additional symbols may be used, however, the meaning of these must be clearly noted on the pedigree.

iii. **Clinical examination:** The examination of patients must be done thoroughly, specially the face, skull, jaw, hair, height of individual, weight, span and body segments. In the systemic examination special attention must be paid to urogenital system, secondary sexual characters and external genitalia, because most of the referred genetic cases are of primary sterility, reproductive failure and ambiguous genitalia.

iv. **Investigations:** The routine simple investigations done in genetic OPD are dermatoglyphic studies and buccal smear for Barr bodies to determine the sex in ambiguous genitalia found in some clinical disorders and genetic syndromes for twin studies, disputed paternity and in population genetics.

Biochemical assays for various enzymes and hormones, etc. are essential for diagnosing inborn errors of metabolism.

Carrier detection tests can also be done by biochemical analysis for a particular substance in X-linked disorders.

Table 9.3: Lag index score to find out frequency in a population

I. Digital Patterns

Ulnar loop (U) Opens to ulnar side	Whorl (W)	Arch (A)	Radial loop (R) opens to radial side

Pattern type : The digit are numbered starting with the thumb as number one. If one of the thumb have an ulnar loop, circle 'UU' under digit 1. etc. Circle one score in each of the five digit groups.

Digit 1 or thumb		Digit 2 index		Digit 3 middle		Digit 4 ring		Digit 5 little finger	
AA, AU, AR, AW	+0.19	UU	+0.61	UU	+0.12	RR, UP	+0.89	RR, RU, RW, RA	+1.42
UU	+0.12	UW, UA, WA	−0.29	WW, WA, WR	−0.17	RA	+0.65	WW, WA	+0.14
UN	−0.10	WW	−0.73	UW	0.29	RW	+0.30	UU, UA	−0.02
WW	−0.30	AA	−0.80	UA, UR	−0.61	AU, AW	+0.23	UW	−0.10
RR, RU, RW	−0.48	RU	−0.84	AA, RR, AR	−0.89	UU	+0.07	AA	−0.37
		RR, RA, RW	−1.54			UW	−0.17		
						WW, AA	−0.24		

Total Score I = _____

Contd...

Table 9.3: Lag index score to find out frequency in a population (*Contd...*)

II. **Palms and Soles:** Circle one score in each of the four groups

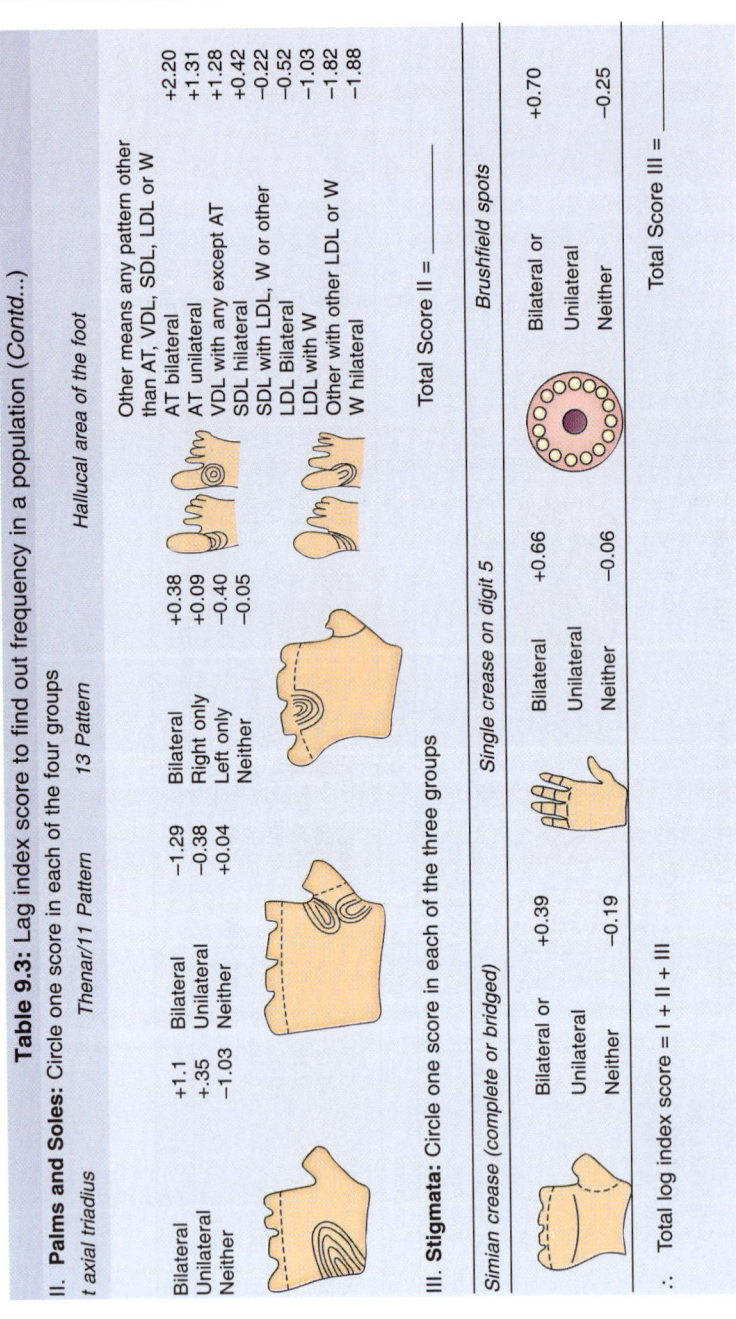

t axial triadius		Thenar/11 Pattern		13 Pattern		Hallucal area of the foot	
Bilateral	+1.1	Bilateral	−1.29	Bilateral	+0.38	Other means any pattern other than AT, VDL, SDL, LDL or W	
Unilateral	+.35	Unilateral	−0.38	Right only	+0.09	AT bilateral	+2.20
Neither	−1.03	Neither	+0.04	Left only	−0.40	AT unilateral	+1.31
				Neither	−0.05	VDL with any except AT	+1.28
						SDL hilateral	+0.42
						SDL with LDL, W or other	−0.22
						LDL Bilateral	−0.52
						LDL with W	−1.03
						Other with other LDL or W	−1.82
						W hilateral	−1.88

Total Score II = _____

III. **Stigmata:** Circle one score in each of the three groups

Simian crease (complete or bridged)		Single crease on digit 5		Brushfield spots	
Bilateral or Unilateral	+0.39	Bilateral	+0.66	Bilateral or Unilateral	+0.70
		Unilateral			
Neither	−0.19	Neither	−0.06	Neither	−0.25

Total Score III = _____

∴ Total log index score = I + II + III = _____

Table 9.4: Summary of unusual dermatoglyphic findings in various syndromes*

	Control	Trisomy 21 (Down)	Trisomy D	Trisomy E	XO (Turner)	4p–	5p–	18p–
Finger patterns								
10 ulnar loops	7.0	4.0	–	0.3	–	–	–	–
> 8 whorls	7.0	0.5	–	<0.3	–	–	4.0	4
> 7 arches	1.7	0.2	9	49.3	–	+	6.0	–
Radial loop on digit 1	0.3	5.0	43	50.0	–	–	3.0	20.0
Radial loop on digit 4 to 5	2.4		21	2.0	–	–	3.0	–
Palmar patterns								
Bilateral t"	3.0	27.0	28	10.0	11	–	–	–
Bilateral 12 pattern	1.0	4.0	–	–				
Bilateral thenar/11	3.0	0.1	11	–	1	15.0	+	–
Bilateral thenar exit to Aline	3.0	0.7	14	3.0	3	+	+	–
Absent a, b, c or d	10.0	1.0	–	+	–	1/5	+	–
Hand creases								
Bilateral simian	2.0	15.0	28	16.0	3	17.0	11	24.0
Sidney	6.0	–	–	–	–	–	–	–
Single 5th finger	0.5	32.0	20	90.0	–	–	–	–
Hallucal patterns								
Tibial arch	0.6	97.0	–	33.0	–	–	–	–
Tibial loop	10.0	0.05	4	1.5	1	–	–	–
Fibular loop under pattern	2.0	–	–	–	–	–	–	–

* The numbers below the syndromes represent the magnitude of the increase over the frequency in controls, e.g. 10 ulnar loops is 4x as frequent in Down's syndrome as in the general population + and – denote an increase or a decrease when precise figures are not available.

Investigative methods for prenatal diagnosis or genetic disorders can be divided into two headings.

a. *Invasive*—aminocentesis, placentocentesis, featoscopy, amniography and fetography.

b. *Non-invasive*—biochemical analysis of maternal and fetal urine, radiography, ultrasonography.

Transabdominal amniocentesis combined with ultrasonography is the most widely used method for prenatal diagnosis. By amniocentesis, the cell free analysis of the amniotic fluid, study of various types of cells or after cultivation of cells is done. There are risks involved in amniocentesis like fetal death, amnionitis, fetal puncture, leakage of amniotic fluid and maternal vaginal bleeding. By ultrasonography on the other hand, being a non-invasive method and thus no risks to fetus or mother, a number of genetic abnormalities can be diagnosed in addition to verification of fetus being alive, determination of gestational age by measuring the head size of fetus, diagnosing the multiple gestations for determining the placental and fetal positions and detecting gross fetal and placental malformations like anencephaly and hydatid mole respectively.

Some abnormalities diagnosed ultrasonographically (prenatally)

- Anencephaly
- Duodenal atresia
- Diaphragmatic hernia
- Encephalocele
- Hydramnios
- Hydrocephalous
- Intrathoracic cyst
- Meningomyelocele
- Oligohydramnios
- Oesophageal atresia
- Omphalocele
- Osteogenesis imperfecta with fractures in utero
- Polycystic kidney
- Renal agenesis

- Short limbs dwarfism
- Small chest wall
- Spina bifida

Karyotyping

The chromatin material in the dividing cell is arrested during metaphase stage when the white blood cells are cultured, because at this stage chromatin material is in its maximum condensed form and individual chromosomes can be visualised on the equator of the spindle. This property has been taken into useful purpose of studying the morphology of chromosomes. The chromosome spread is stained and photographed. From the photograph, the chromosomes spread is arranged in height and position of centromere and photographed again for detailed study. Thus, a karyotype can be defined as a set of chromosomes arranged in a standard classification form a photomicrograph of the metaphase spread.

Evaluation

The evaluation of an inherited disease has to be done considering the fact that an individual's phenotype is the result of an interaction between the genotype and the lifetime environment. The family history to determine the inheritance pattern is evaluated as follows.

i. **Autosomal dominant inheritance:** Implies a single gene expressing without regard to the other gene at a particular locus and as per McKusick (1968), there are more than 700 dominant or suspected dominant diseases known. In the family history, the criteria suggesting this type of inheritance are:

   a. Each generation shows affected members, i.e. no skipping
   b. Unaffected individuals do not transmit the trait to their offsprings.
   c. The affected individuals transmit the trait to about 50% of their offsprings.
   d. Both males and females have equal chances of getting the trait.

ii. **Autosomal recessive inheritance:** Implies a pair of genes are required for expression and the individual is known as a carrier when such single gene is present and trait is not expressed. In the family history, the criteria for such type of inheritance are:

   a. The disease is seen in sibs, i.e. brothers and sisters and not in parents or offsprings.

   b. Consanguinity of parents is almost always there as regards the affected individual.

   c. If both the parents are carrier, there are chances of 25% offsprings to be affected.

   d. Males and females are equally affected.

iii. **Sex-linked inheritance:** Practically, an X-linked because the Y-chromosome in males has only known genes for hairly pinna and H and Y antigen. The overall incidence of X-linked disorder is 0.5 per thousand. The females are carriers of only one gene, not expressing is present while in the males, the one gene on only one X-chromosome is said to be in hemizygous state and will always express itself (Refer to Fig. 7.2).

   1. *X-linked dominant inheritance:* Implies a single gene present on X-chromosome in females may be in homo- or heterozygous state while in males, gene is always in heterozygous state. The family history will have the following criteria.

      a. Females are affected twice as commonly as males.

      b. Affected males transmit the trait to all his daughters but none to his sons.

      c. When an affected male marries an affected homozygous female, all the children will be affected, and the daughters being homozygous.

      d. When an affected male marries an affected heterozygous female, all the daughters and half the sons will be affected.

      e. When a normal male marries an affected homozygous female all the children will be affected, the daughters being heterozygous.

f. When a normal male marries an affected heterozygous female, half the children both daughters and sons, would be affected, and daughters becoming heterozygous.

Thus X-linked dominant disorders follow the same pattern as autosomal dominant disorders. (Refer to pedigree charts in Figs 7.1 to 7.5)

2. *X-linked recessive inheritance:* Implies a recessive gene present on one X-chromosome in males will always express as there is no gene present for contrasting traits, there being no other X-chromosome, while the females being carrier the trait is not expressed. The family history will have the following criteria.

a. Only males are affected except in some rare cases.

b. From pedigree the disease may appear to skip one or more generations and affected males are always related through carrier females.

c. On an average about 50% of sons of a carrier female are affected.

Thus in families, where there is only one affected member or when there is limited family history available, for evaluation following points must be considered.

i. Whether the clinical picture is resembling with the previously described genetic disease exhibiting autosomal recessive or sex-linked recessive inheritance.

ii. Whether the clinical picture is the result of some environmental or developmental insult and thus not hereditary.

iii. Whether the clinical picture represents a new mutation, which might have occured in the germinal line of either the unaffected parent or in the genome of the zygote.

A new mutation may follow a previously described pattern of inheritance for the observed clinical condition or it may be a different locus to have different pattern of inheritance. The laboratory techniques becoming more sophisticated, it will be possible to detect the presence of recessive genes in the heterozygous state.

Some cases with genotype of a specific disease fail to express any clinical features of the disease due to *reduced penetrance* thus having an all or nothing phenomenon as regards the detection of disease.

Most of the genetic diseases also show *variable expressivity* and *genetic heterogeneity*.

Abnormal sex ratio and variable age of onset are other setbacks for evaluation of a genetic disease.

Most continuously disturbed traits like height, weight and intelligence do not follow the simple Mendelian pattern of inheritance because a number of genes are responsible for small and similar cumulative effects known as *multifactorial polygenic* or *quantitative effects*. The characteristics of a polygenic inheritance are:

  i. the rarer the trait in the population, greater the risk to relatives, and greater difference in risk between first and second degree relatives and between second and third degree relatives.

 ii. the more severe the malformation in the proband case, the greater the risk to relatives.

iii. if there is a sex difference in frequency of the trait, risks will be higher to relatives of affected members of the less frequently affected sex.

 iv. if there is another affected relative of proband case, there will be higher risk to other relatives.

In addition to detailed family history, which is valuable in multifactorial inheritance, the diagnosis of all affected or reportedly affected members within the family is important from all able sources so as to establish a specific diagnosis. The degree of relationship amongst the various affected members must also be clearly established. Special attention should be paid to the similarity of the phenotypic expression among the various affected relatives and lastly, relevant prenatal and postnatal environmental factors should be obtained.

Most of chromosomal abnormalities can be diagnosed after the careful study of karyotype, e.g. Down's, Turner's, Kilnefelter's syndromes, etc. Some of the disorders can be diagnosed by special banding patterns. Specifically for deletions, inversions, translocations etc. Genetic markers like blood groups, DNA markers, HLA system, immunoglobulins studies can lead to diagnosis of disputed paternity, determination of zygosity in twins, illegitimacy of child, compatibility for organ transplantation, etc.

Prenatal diagnosis of some of the inherited disorders can be achieved by a number of methods as follows.

i. **Aminocentesis:** 15–16 week of pregnancy is the ideal time because by this time sufficient amount of fluid can be withdrawn for culture as well as biochemical analysis. While doing this procedure, the various hazards of the said procedure must be kept in mind like abortions, perinatal problems like respiratory distress and congenital talipes and dislocation of hip, etc.

ii. **Ultrasound:** This method is also ancillary to aminocentasis in localization of placenta and detects conditions like anencephaly, spina bifida, microcephaly, congenital heart disease and intrauterine growth retardation. The approximate age of the developing fetus with expected date of delivery can also be estimated by this method.

iii. **Fetoscopy (amnioscopy):** Usually done during 18–22 weeks of pregnancy for detection of malformation of limbs or digits, face like ear and cleft palate, malformation of genetalia and spine. Recently fetoscopic, i.e. fetal skin biopsy is done to diagnose epidermosis bullosa.

iv. **Fetal blood sampling:** Which can be done either indirectly by placental aspiration or directly the blood withdrawn from root of umbilical cord with the help of a fetoscope. The blood samples are used to diagnose the inborn blood disorders like thalassaemia, sickle cell anaemia, and haemophylia, etc.

v. **Radiographic methods:** Usually done during mid-trimester or about 20–22nd week of pregnancy, by either amniography for visualisation of fetus by constrast, and for conditions like hydramnios, achondrogenesis, gastrointestinal atresias, diaphragmatic hernia, etc. or by fetography to diagnose some major anamolies that manifest externally like limb length anamolies, and other anamolies like anencephaly, meningomyelocoele, etc.

vi. **Maternal serum and urine analysis:** Serum sampling is usually done during 16–18 weeks of pregnancy. Raised α-fetoprotein levels are indicative of neural tube defect in fetus. If a repeat sample also shows elevated levels, ultrasonography and aminocenta should be done to confirm the diagnosis. Similarly, urine sampling though less reliable than serum as a diagnostic tool, does help in analysing an abnormality.

III. GENETIC COUNSELLING

In late fifties, most of the nonmedical geneticists were recognised to give advise to human beings as a side line to their main research and teaching genetics of animals and plants and their counselling consisted mainly in applying the Mandelian laws to a particular family faced with the problem of genetic origin. Much of the information about the inheritance of human diseases was misleading, because of the tendency to choose strikingly familial cases. There were few textbooks available in human genetics and none for genetic counselling. There has been tremendous growth in the knowledge of human genetics making the task of a genetic counsellor more difficult.

The present medical geneticist is a physician specialising in human genetics and is required to give advise to a patient or the family as a whole or to even entire government on matter pertaining to the causation, incidence, and risks of inherited diseases to recur. The importance of a genetic counsellor in the fields of radiation hazards, drugs induced and mutant viral strains induced hazards is going to be increased and thus in a medical institution for teaching the geneticist is going to be the key figure. Genetic counselling is thus defined as the branch which deals with the problem of giving advise to families suffering or likely to suffer from a genetic disorder and give the proper line of treatment after establishing the proper diagnosis. The counselling is done for immediate preventive and social health promotional measures in genetic disorders. The counseling, however, depends mainly on the accurate diagnosis and definition of aetiology and the mode of inheritance. The course and prognosis of the disorder must be evaluated on the basis of family history from pedigree charting, appropriate tests, to estimate the recurrence risk is made. After making the decision, the appropriate line of action is decided only with the concurrence of family. Decisions to be taken are as follows:

• Whether to go for the marriage or not
• Whether to have another baby or not
• Whether to use contraceptive measures, or seek sterilization
• Whether to adopt a child
• Have antenatal diagnosis done
• Have therapeutic abortion

Genetic screening programmes to identify individuals with treatable genetic diseases, and couples at higher risk of getting children with severe genetic diseases are an important element of genetic counselling programmes. But added to this, there are some legal, moral and ethical issues to be dealt carefully by the geneticist. The problems can arise during mistaken paternity, i.e. rarely in Tay-Sachs disease or PKU when the proband is homozygous for an allele while it is present only in carrier mother or in sickle cell anaemia, the allele is present only in proband being absent in both the parents, discovered accidently during routine blood group testing. Similarly the problem of confidentiality for a serious genetic disorder in the family as to inform whom regarding the diagnosed disorder. In the United States, the laws governing the confidentiality are being introduced. Lastly, some national ethical issues like the fundamental right of parents to produce a defective child, which will be a burden for the family and indirectly for the nation or the right of the defective offspring to be born if viable or the rights of a fetus in the society, the legal problems arising after the birth of a defective child.

IV. EXPERIMENTAL GENETICS AND EUGENETICS

The understanding of human genetics has mainly been derived from experiments on micro-organisms and laboratory animals, humans being ill suited for experimental work. For this two factors have helped a lot:

i. That the genetic material DNA is almost of same the composition in all living organisms and,

ii. That the genetic material can be manipulated in and in between various living forms.

Because of the above two factors, the selective breeding of desirable traits in plants and animals for improvement is as old as civilization, and this knowledge is being applied to benefit the human beings as well, recently. The evolutionary destiny of all living organisms is dependent on genetic constitution and environment beyond their control. Human beings alone are able to control their environment and to some extent their genetic constitution. Thus, the biological evolution can be compared with the cultural evolution in some aspects as shown in Table 9.5.

The important experimental work started from Mendel's experiments on garden peas laying the foundation of genetic studies.

Studies experimentally in *Dorsophila melanogester* by Morgan and his collaborators helped in understanding the Mendelian laws, linkage, sex determination, crossing over, mutations, multiple alleles and chromosomal mapping, etc.

Experimental studies in Neurospora for recombination and crossing over in mouse somatic cells for details of genetic linkage, in microbes for molecular genetics have greatly added to the knowledge of genetic.

Experiments have proved the DNA to be the genetic material, which is transferred from one generation to another. It was furthered by experiments to give the detailed molecular structure of DNA, genetic code was cracked and synthetic artificial genes could be produced resembling the human genome. The upcoming branch of genetics known *eugenetics* is speedily progressing for the betterment of mankind.

The study of molecular structure of eukaryotic genes can be done by restriction endonuclease analysis, southern hybridization, recombinant DNA cloning and DNA

Table 9.5: A comparison between biological and cultural evolutions

S.no.	Criteria	Biological evolution	Cultural evolution
1	Treated by	Genes	Thoughts
2	Rate of change	Slow	Rapid and exponential,
3	Agents of change selection	Random variation (mutation) and selection	Usually purposeful directional variation
4	Nature of the new variant	Often harmful	Often beneficial
5	Transmission	Parents to offsprings by many means	Wide dissemination
6	Distribution in nature	All forms of life	Unique in humans
7	Interaction requires cultural evolution	Human biology	Human culture requires biological evolution
8	Complexity achieved	Rare formation of new genes by duplication	Frequent formation of new ideas and technologies

sequencing. All these experimental works in genetic engineering are gaining popularity.

GENE THERAPY

The concept of introducing a foreign DNA sequence having a stable integration, gene expression and proper regulation in the target organ started in 1979, when a 25 years old student of Stanford University, USA, experimented on a deadly virus by taking out its gene (a single gene) for replication and instead replaced with rabbit's gene for haemoglobin and such viruses loaded within rabbit's gene were implanted on kidney cells of monkey and cultured and surprisingly, the chains of haemoglobin molecules were formed, thus beginning the era of gene therapy. The therapy involves replacement of a defective/deficient/abnormal gene into the cells of a patient with a normal gene product. Following criteria must be fulfilled before the therapy can be started:

   i. Formulation of a governing body for regulating the techniques, therapeutic and safety aspects of gene therapy.

ii. Gene delivery mechanism is done by two method, i.e. *Ex-vivo* or *in-vitro* transfer methods are used for transfer of gene after removing the cells of patient and introducing appropriate DNA sequence in these cells which are transplanted back into patients, while with *in-vivo* approach, the desired DNA sequence is introduced in the target organ.

Techniques used for gene transfer

a. *Physical* or *nonviral gene delivery system*

- DNA transfer via liposome is known as liposome mediated gene therapy. This method has the advantage of transferring large amount of DNA sequences into the target cell and such large amount of DNA can be compared to an artificial mini-chromosome responsible for regulation of gene expression in a controlled and physiological manner. The disadvantage of cell transfer is that its expression is short lived and thus requires repetition of therapy. The method liposome mediated gene therapy is being actively used in cases of cystic fibrosis patients in UK and USA.

- Second physical method is known as receptor mediated endocytosis, i.e. targeted nonviral gene delivery system. In this method, a complex of plasmid DNA containing foreign DNA and specific polypeptide ligands for which the cell has receptor is targeted recalling endocytosis→fusion with liposome→degrading of complex→foreign genome from liposome to be expressed. The rate of escape of foreign DNA from lyposome can be increased by inclusion of adenovirus or fusogenic gene products. These nonviral techniques include direct micro-infection, electroporation, calcium phosphate and plasmid and liposome based gene transfer.

b. *Biological or viral transfer Method*

In this technique viral vectors are used for an efficient mode of delivery upto target cells. Various viruses used are retrovirus, adenovirus, herpes virus, adenovirus associated virus or parvovirus, etc. The viruses are made replication deficient by removing encapsidation gene sequences.

The advantages and disadvantages of the biological methods of transfer vary according to the virus used but in general they can be listed as follows.

Advantages of such a viral transfer method over the non-viral methods are:

- 100% transduction is possible.
- Packaging cell lines have been created for infecting a variety of host ranges.
- There is no lysis of cell after infection.
- The transferred genes can integrate precisely at the cellular DNA.

Disadvantages of viral transfer methods are:

- They cannot be started as replication defective recombination viruses.
- Sometimes even replication deficient virus can kill the target cell.

  Thus, all viruses used have advantages and disadvantages of their own. But till date, retroviruses enclose a RNA molecule which is for suppressing the varieties of malignant neoplasms, adenovirus having double helix DNA is being engineered for detecting nervous system tumour and adeno associated virus having small DNA virus, always required help of adenovirus to be replicated to herpes virus—a long DNA virus has been worked to suppress nervous system therapy.

- *Expression:* The next criterion for gene therapy is appropriate expression of new gene in which the target cell is produced. This is one of the biggest challenges in gene therapy for enhancing level of gene expression. Thus controlled and elevated level of transcription is the fundamental requirement of any gene transfer protocol.

- *Safety:* The fourth criterion for transfer of level genes into the cells must not harm the cell and in extension the organisation.
- *Ethical aspect* is the next context for gene therapy especially a germ based gene therapy as therapeutic gene cells may be based to damage further generation.

  The negative application of gene therapy are so frightening that regulation will have the strength planned before making the technology public.
- *Conclusion:* Gene therapy may become a useful asset for treating before threatening diseases but may not wholly replace the currently practiced problems.

The target tissues in animated kingdoms are liver, muscle, CNS, bone marrow, and the target cells are fibroblasts entitled bias cells, epithelial cells, gene cells, etc.

Diseases accommodate to gene therapy are cancer, periferal vascular disease, coronary artery disease, AIDS, etc.

These are genes present on DNA and RNA of humans and animals respectively, responsible for tumours in different chromosomes in human beings and animals.

Normal mammalian cell contains DNA sequences homologous to viral oncogenes which are cell proto-oncogenes or cellular oncogenes.

GENETICS OF CANCER IN HUMAN

The relationship of cancer and human chromosome started in 1902, when Prof Theodor Brang (Germany) stated a change in one chromosome may be starting part of cancer. It has made 50 years to subsidize his theory when in 1959, Peter-C Mowell and David A Huggford discovered philadelphia chromosome associated with mycloid leukaemia in chromosome 9. It is thought that the chromosomes carrying oncogenes can be dealt for malignant transformation.

Cancer is thought to be having a distorted cell cycle with defects at Gap1 leading to defects in synthesis and Gap 2 and thus the mitotic phase. Two check points have been seen to detect DNA damage phase.

i. At Gap1—synthesis transition
ii. At Gap 2—mitosis transition

In Gap 1 leading to the synthesis of P53, a tumour suppressor gene guards the cell at Gap 1 leading to synthesise boundary.

Abnormality of P53 gene increases aneuploidy and gene amplification. Thus, leading the cell towards malignancy. In cancer susceptible syndrome, ataxia telonglectasis cells defective for P53 continue to enter S phase after irradiation and thus enhanced chances of getting breast cancer.

Gap 2—mitosis, suggests the nonregulation of cellular traffic or that may result in cancer of pancreas and activation of C-mos protoncogenes.

EXERCISE

1. Define the following.
   a. Population genetics
   b. Genetic counselling
   c. Dermatoglyphics
   d. Experimental genetics.
2. Explian Hardy–Weinberg rule.
3. Write short notes on:
   a. Genetic drift
   b. Genetic heterogeneity
   c. Multiple births in genetics
   d. Blood group chimera.
4. Write notes on:
   a. Finger tip patterns
   b. Triradius
   c. Log index score.
5. How a genetic disorder is assessed for genetic counselling? Enumerate the methods and investigations required.
6. Enumerate the methods used to diagnose genetic disorder prenatally.

7. Fill in the blanks.
   a. The genetic material is .... almost of ....
      composition in all .... organisms.
   b. Genetic material can be .... in and in between
      various .... forms.
   c. Selective .... of desirable traits in .... and
      .... for improvement is as old as civilization.
   d. The study of molecular .... of eukaryotic ....
      can be done by restriction .... analysis, southern
      .... recombinant .... cloning and
      sequencing.

10

Common Genetic Disorders

According to Fraser Roberts (1970), the incidence of serious developmental abnormalities is 1:30 in each pregnancy appearing early in life. Whereas, Emery (1974), stated that roughly 20 children admitted in hospital have a disorder which is entirely genetic in origin, either a single gene disorder or chromosomal abnormality. Multifactorial disorders with prominent genetic element accounts for 15% of pediatrics and 11% of adults in patients.

Each single mutant gene exhibits one of the four patterns of Mendelian inheritance.

   i. Autosomal recessive

  ii. Autosomal dominant

 iii. X-linked recessive

 iv. X-linked dominant

The multifactorial disorders are given in Chapter 7 under modes of inheritance as far as single gene defects are concerned, and chromosomal defects are given in Table 7.4 with some clinical features including those of sex chromosomes.

DOWN SYNDROME

Statistically, the incidence is 1:800 live births and twice amongst all conceptus, but more than half of trisomy-21 fetuses are spontaneously aborted during early pregnancy. There is high correlation between advanced maternal age. About 90% of karyotypically abnormal conceptions do not survive pregnancy. In live births about half are due to autosomes and other half due to sex chromosomes (Figs 10.1 to 10.3).

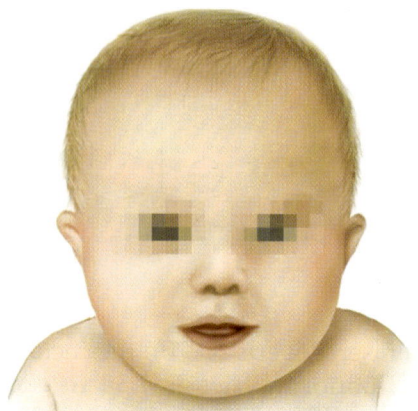

Fig. 10.1: Trisomy 21

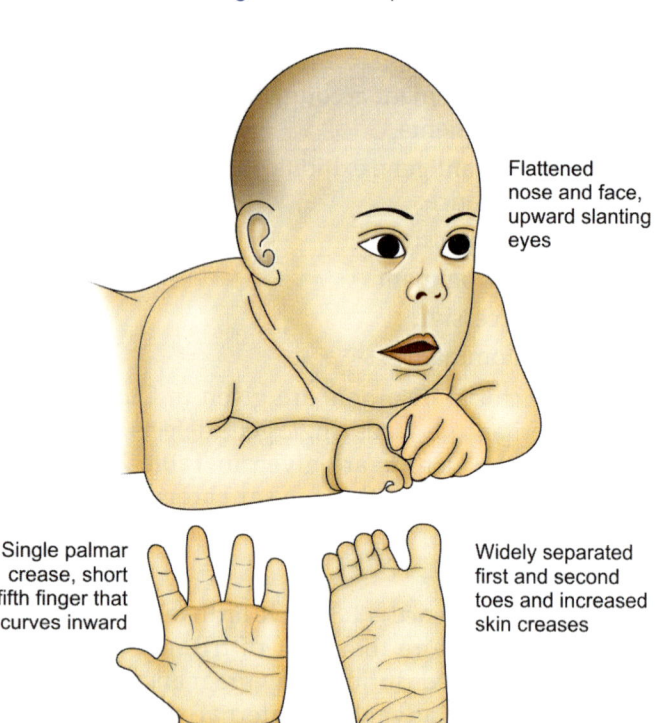

Flattened
nose and face,
upward slanting
eyes

Single palmar
crease, short
fifth finger that
curves inward

Widely separated
first and second
toes and increased
skin creases

Fig. 10.2: Trisomy 13

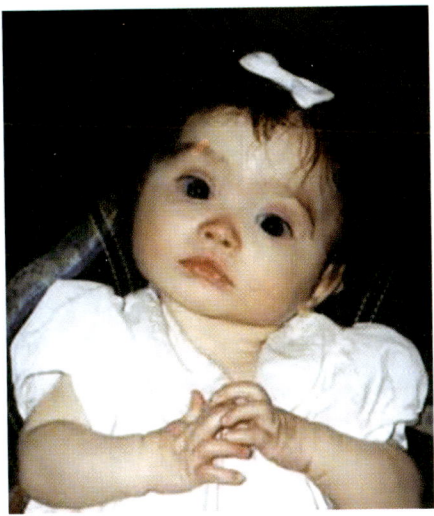

Fig. 10.3: Trisomy 18 (mental retardation)

A high correlation exists between advanced maternal age and non-dysjunction resulting in the presence of an extra chromosome in the offspring, the reason is unknown. It can be due to aging of oocyte living in suspended animation during meiotic division from late fetal life, till its participation in ovulation.

Heteromorphism of parental origin of non-dysjunction due to abnormal segregation is found in about 10–20% of cases. The recurrence risk of trisomy to chromosomally normal parents is uncertain.

Translocation Down Syndrome

Ninty-five per cent cases of Down's syndrome are due to translocation and centric fusion between chromosomes 21 and 13, 14 and 15. About 1% are mosaic, minimally as some mosaics remain undetected particularly among phenotypically normal parents of trisomic offsprings, remaining are due to translocation. Clinical features are compared in a tabulated form for the most common autosomal trisomic syndromes in Table 10.1.

Table 10.1: Clinical features of the most common autosomal trisomy syndromes

Dermatoglyphic patterns and flexion creases	Trisomic syndrome on chromosome number	Clinical features
Ulnar loops on all fingers, radial loops on fingers 4 and 5. Distal axial triradius or large AID angle on palms. Arch tibial or small loop distal in hallucal area on soles. Simian crease; single crease on finger 5.	21 Trisomy	Mental retardation, hypotonia. Flat occiput, oblique palpebral fissure, epicanthic folds (Fig. 10.1), brush field spots in iris, protruding tongue, prominent malformed ears, flat nasal bridge. Septal defects of heart specially of endocardial cushions. Decreased acetabular and iliac angles. Small penis, cryptorchidism. Simian crease, gap between 1st and 2nd toes (Fig. 10.2). High arched palate, strabismus, short neck, small teeth, furrowed tongue, intestinal atresia, imperforate anus and Hirschsprung's disease.
Arches on fingers and toes. Single crease on finger 5 or on all fingers.	18 Trisomy	Mental retardation (Fig. 10.3), hypotonia, failure to thrive, and low birth weight. Prominent occiput, micrognathia, low set malformed ears. VSD and PDA short sternum, diaphragmatic hernia, horse shoe kidney, small pelvis, limited abduction of hip, inguinal and/or umbilical hernia. Flexion deformity of fingers, short dorsiflexed big toes, rocker bottom feet, and rarely phocomelia. Cleft lip and cleft palate, ocular anamolies, simian crease, hypoplasia of

Contd...

Table 10.1: Clinical features of the most common autosomal trisomy syndromes (*Contd...*)

Dermatoglyphic patterns and flexion creases	Trisomic syndrome on chromosome number	Clinical features
		fingernails, widely spaced nipples, webbed neck, single umbilical artery and tracheo-oesophageal fistula.
Distal axial triradius or large ATD angle. Arch fibular or arch fibular-S in hallucal area. Simian crease.	13 Trisomy	Mental retardation, failure to thrive, capillary heamangiomas persistent, fetal haemoglobin seizures, apneic episodes.
		Microcephally, cleft lip and palate, midline scalp defects, microphthalmia, colobomata, low set malformed ears, apparent deafness.
		Congenital heart disease mainly septal defects PDA. Polycystic kidneys, bicornuate uterus, cryptorchidism. Polydactyl hyperconvex or hypoplastic fingernails, simian crease.
		Flexion deformity of fingers, single umbilical artery, shallow supraorbital ridges, micrognathia, retroflexible thumb, rocker bottom feet, omphalocele.

Trisomy Involving Other Chromosomes

The accurate recognition of individual chromosomes has led to the identification of new autosomal trisomy syndromes for chromosomes 8 and 9 and some other, but documentation for other chromosomes except 8 and 9 is still lacking. Trisomy, virtually for every autosome has been documented in the products of early spontaneous abortions, i.e. full trisomy is probably lethal. Partial trisomy due to duplication or duplication deficiency for almost all autosomes produced by translocation or inversion have been reported.

Adrenogenital Syndrome (Congenital Adrenal Hyperplasia)

This condition is produced by congenital adrenal hyperplasia and by virilizing adrenocortical tumours. When congenital, it is caused by an inborn defect in the biosynthesis of adrenal cortisol. Usually five levels of enzymetic defects are known as shown below.

Mineralocorticoids	Glucocorticoids	Sex hormones
Cholesterol ↓	17-Hydroxy	Dehydro-EPI
Pregnenolone ↓	Pregnenolone →	Androsterone (DMA)
Progesterone →	17-Hydroxy 11-Deoxy cortisol (Compound S) ↓	Progesterone
	Cortisol (Compound F)	

Deficiency of 21-hydroxylase accounts for 95% of affected patients. The enzyme is a cytochrome-P450 enzyme, located on the short arm of chromosome 6, within the HLA complex and is closely linked to HLA-B and C4A and C4B complement genes. Two classic forms of disease, saltwasting and simple virilizing are described. It occurs in every 1 in 5000 births approximately. The particular enzyme defect and its degree is genetically determined, usually being inherited as an autosomal recessive trait with clinical expression in the homozygous state. Females are more often affected than males, and the age at which the disorder first menifests depends on the completeness and nature of the enzyme defect. If the enzyme deficiency is severe, excess androgen secretion occurring in utero, leads to the birth of a female child with an enlarged clitoris, variable fusion of labia and a rudimentary vagina that may not open to exterior Fig. 10.4a.

In some, a complete penile urethera is seen. The child is thus a pseudohermaphrodite having ovaries but no testicular tissue in gonads. The male child with congenital adrenal hyperplasia may show precocious development of external genetalia at or soon after birth is marked by enzyme deficiency and the

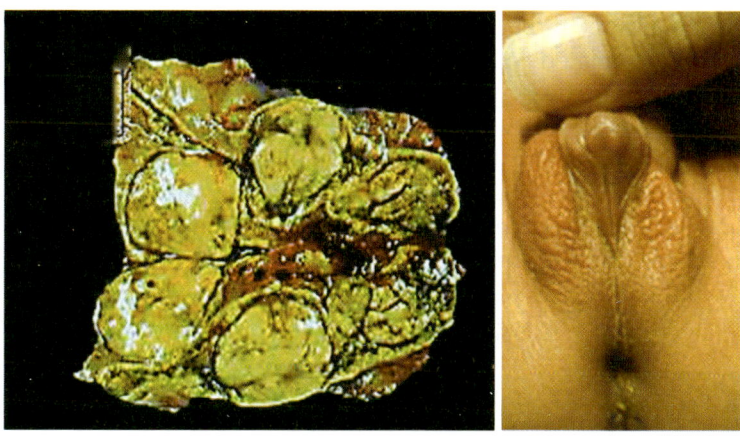

Fig. 10.4a

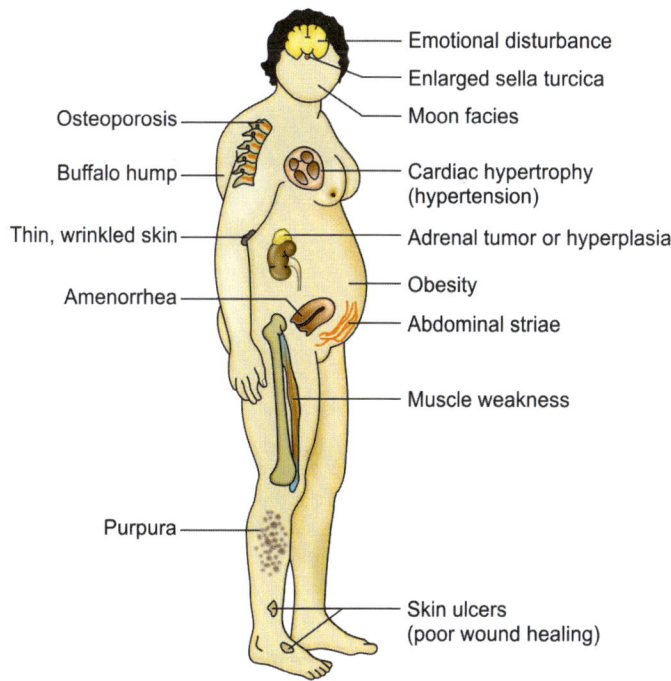

Osteoporosis

Buffalo hump

Thin, wrinkled skin

Amenorrhea

Purpura

Emotional disturbance

Enlarged sella turcica

Moon facies

Cardiac hypertrophy
(hypertension)

Adrenal tumor or hyperplasia

Obesity

Abdominal striae

Muscle weakness

Skin ulcers
(poor wound healing)

Fig. 10.4b

prognosis of child becomes grave if the defect is not diagnosed early and treated. With lesser degree of enzyme deficiency the clinical features appear late. Male child presents with precocious puberty and female child has enlarged clitoris, hirsutism and acne. Both sexes have increased skeletal growth and muscular development. Girls have primary amenorrhoea and lack of secondary sexual characteristics (Fig. 10.4b). Boys have testicular atrophy leading to infertility but the secondary sexual characteristics are within normal limits or exaggerated by increased androgen secretion.

Cri-Du-Chat Syndrome

It is named so because the cry of the child resembles that of a kitten and is characterised by high pitched tense phonation. It is a structural abnormality in chromosome 5 by a deletion in the short arm. The typical cry of the infant, however, tends to disappear in late infancy, and similar cry may be noted in some mentally retarded children (Fig. 10.5).

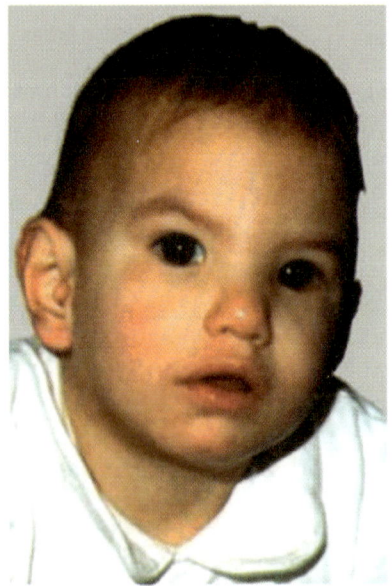

Fig. 10.5: Microcephaly antimongoloid small palpebral fissure

The deletion in short arm of chromosome 4 are severely malformed and retarded and do not have the typical cry. Some important clinical signs (*see* Table 6.1). A number of these deletion syndromes may show ring chromosomes due to deletion at both ends of chromosome.

Turner's Syndrome

About 55% of cases are due to complete monosomy of X with a karyotype 45X. The frequency being 1:10000 live female births, as noted in a small proportion of conceptuses. 45X karyotype is one of the most common type seen amongst the spontaneous aborted products and the only well documented monosomy in human. The X-chromosome is maternal in 77% and paternal in 23% cases. The mechanism of origin is uncertain and not influenced by maternal age. The seasonal effect is probable because non-dysjunction occurs in about two thirds of births during the months between May and October. Mosaicism (46 XX/45 X) is seen in 25% of cases and only 5% to 10% are complete monosomy of 45X are live births. Other types of mosaics like isochromosome for long arm, deletion of short arm and rings of X-chromosomes are much less common and the cases used to be diagnosed only at puberty or childhood which fail to achieve sexual maturation. In newborns the typical lymphoedema of hands and feet (Fig. 10.6), on dorsum is a characteristic feature along with webbing of neck (Fig. 10.7) low posterior hair line (Fig. 10.8), small mandible, prominent ears, epitanthic folds, high arched palate, broad chest giving a false widely spaced nipples, cubitus valgum and hyperconvex finger nails, height below 3rd percentile. In mosaics, the abnormalities are a few. Usually the affected newborn has no characteristic features like oedema but short stature may be the only feature seen. Chromosomal analysis should be done in all suspected cases. A small number of cases with features resembling Turner syndrome have a Y-chromosome, their management being different than monosomy or mosaics. Plasma levels of gonadotrophins specifically of follicular stimulating hormone are elevated in children above 10 years of age. Radiological studies may show cardiovascular or renal abnormalities. The

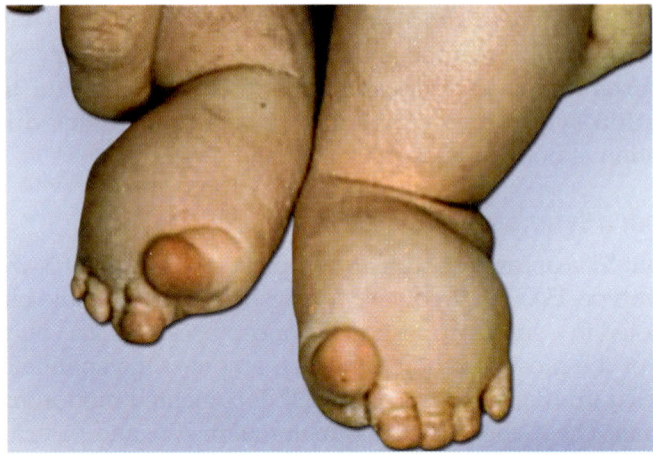

Fig. 10.6: Turner's syndrome (lymphoedema of hands and feet)

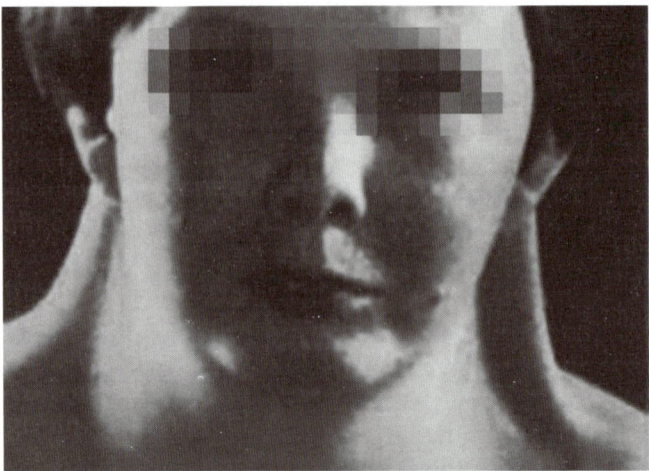

Fig. 10.7: Turner's syndrome for webbing of neck

important skeletal abnormality is shortening of 4th metatarsal or metacarpal bone, epiphyseal dysgenesis in joints of knee and elbow, scoliosis, spina bifida and inadequate mineralization. Mild diabetes (chemical) is seen in about one-third of cases. A high percentage of cases and other family members have significant titers of antithyroid antibodies.

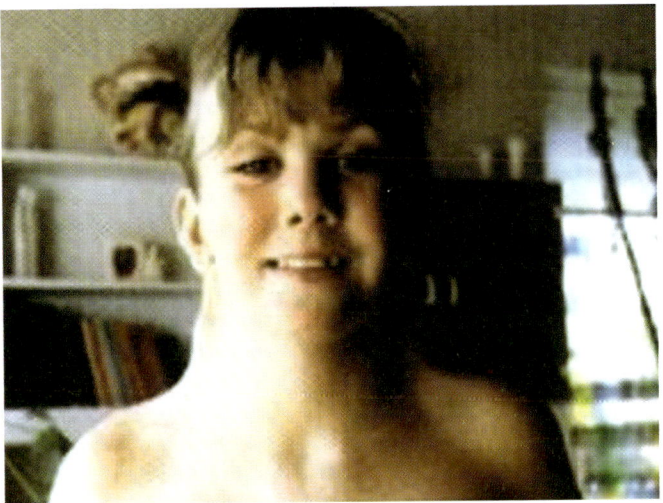

Fig. 10.8: Turner's syndrome with low posterior hairline

Klinefelter or XXY Syndrome

One in 750 newborn males have a 47 XXY karyotype and thus more common than Down's syndrome. It is due to meiotic non-dysjunction of X-chromosome during parental gametogenesis, the extra X-chromosome being maternal in origin in 67% and paternal in 33% cases.

The diagnosis is usually made at the time of puberty (Fig. 10.9). During childhood, before the defects in sexual development, the cases are mentally retarded, anxious, immature, excessively shy or aggressive, tall, slim and underweight having cryptorchidism and/or hypospadias, need to be investigated for this syndrome. About 40% have gynecomastia, sparse facial hair, azoospermia and infertility are associated features at adult age.

The mosaic Klinefelter and variants are not different from the classical form but the severity and frequency of features is diminished and they have better prognosis for virilization, fertility and psychosomatic adjustments. The rare variant 49 XX XY can be detected in childhood because of distinctive features of severe retardation, large malformed ears, a short

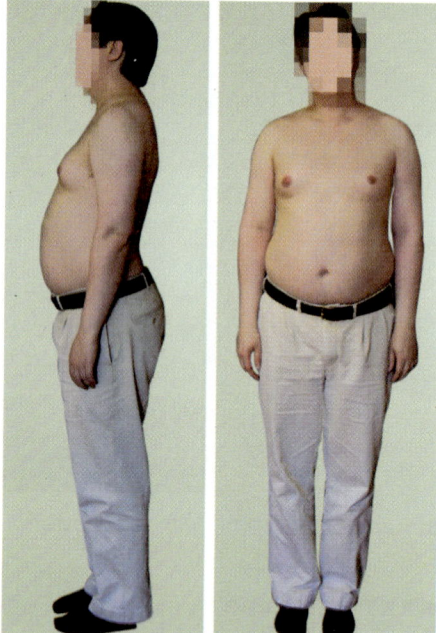

Fig. 10.9: Klinefelter syndrome

neck and atypical facies with wide set eyes having a Mongoloid slant, epicanthus strabismus, a wide flat upturned nose and a large open mouth.

The mosaic and variants having patterns like 46, XY/47, XXY, 46XY/48XXYY, 45X/46XY/46XXY and rarer 48XXXY, 49XXXYY, 50XXXXYY, 47XXY/48 XXXY and so on, it is noteworthy that the Y chromosome determines the male phenotype inspite of having as many as for X chromosomes. XX males have also been reported in about 2:20,0000 males, the male determining genes being translocated from Y-chromosome to X-chromosome during meiosis in father.

Fragile X Syndrome

The most common heritable fragile sites occur on the lone arm of X-chromosome (band g 27-28) and is associated with mental retardation, with or without macro-orchidism in males. The syndrome may account for about 30% of X-linked mental

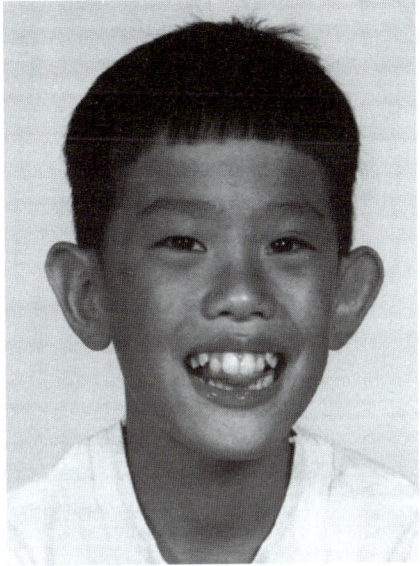

Fig. 10.10: Fragile X syndrome

retardation in males and about 10% of all mild mentally retarded females. The fragile site acts as a chromosomal marker (Fig. 10.10).

Congenital Hypothyroidism (Cretinism)

A condition resulting from deficiency of thyroid hormone during fetal or early neonatal life. The characteristic features being retarded growth and development particularly affecting the skeletal and central nervous system.

Cretinism may be seen as sporadic or endemic forms. Endemic form is seen in areas with severe iodine deficiency and the mother of affected child will have goiter. Sporadic form is rare and is due to athyreosis or failure of embryonic gland to descend in neck. Thyroid deficiency may arise due to partial or complete absence of one of the several enzymes required for biosynthesis of thyroid hormones. In rare cases of dyshormonogenesis, cretinism is associated with goiter, it is often an hereditary familial disorder, sometimes associated with other congenital defects such as deafness (Penderd's

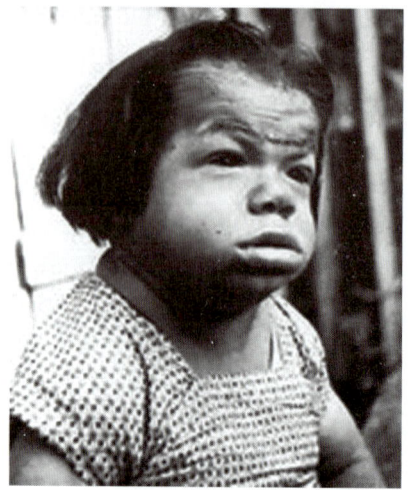

Fig. 10.11: Hypothyroidism (congenital)

syndrome). Thyroid deficiency may occur in fetuses of hyperthyroid mothers on large doses of antithyroid drugs which cross the placental barrier.

The child is lethargic, falls asleep during feeding, fails to thrive and is constipated. The typical facies being broad and puffy flat nose, thickened lips and nostrils enlarged protruding tongue (Fig. 10.11). The abdomen is protruding and associated with umbilical hernia, skin is dry, thickened and sallow, voice is hoarse, hair dark in colour, eyes wideset, dentition is delayed and overall, the child is mentally retarded. Diagnosis can be confirmed by raised serum levels of TSH. Rarely cretinism may be confused with mongolism.

Craniosynostosis

Premature closure of one or more sutures of skull leading to deformity in head and thus damage to brain or eyes depending upon the suture involved. Congenital craniosynostosis originates during embryonic life for unknown reasons. In acquired, it may be associated with rickets, hypophosphatasia, and idiopathic hypercalcaemia and may also occur after shunt operation for hydrocephalus.

When sagittal sutures close prematurely, it leads to scaphoce-phaly, and closure of coronal sutures leads to severe deformity of head (Fig. 10.12) as oxycephaly and acrocephaly with deformity of face and eyes. The roof of orbit being depressed leads to exophthalmos and there may be strabismus, papilloedema, optic atrophy and loss of vision. Complications will be more severe when complete coronal suture and other sutures are also involved. Other malformations such as cardiac defects, choanal atresia, defects of knee and elbow joints, the commonest associated anamoly being syndactyly. A familial form of premature closure of coronal sutures with haemolytic jaundice has been reported. Apert's syndrome (acrocephalo-syndactyly), an autosomal dominant transmitted condition and Carpenter syndrome (acrocephalopoly syndacylt), an autosomal recessive transmitted condition. Crouzon disease, (craniofacial dysostosis) is characterized by acrocephaly, beak shaped nose,

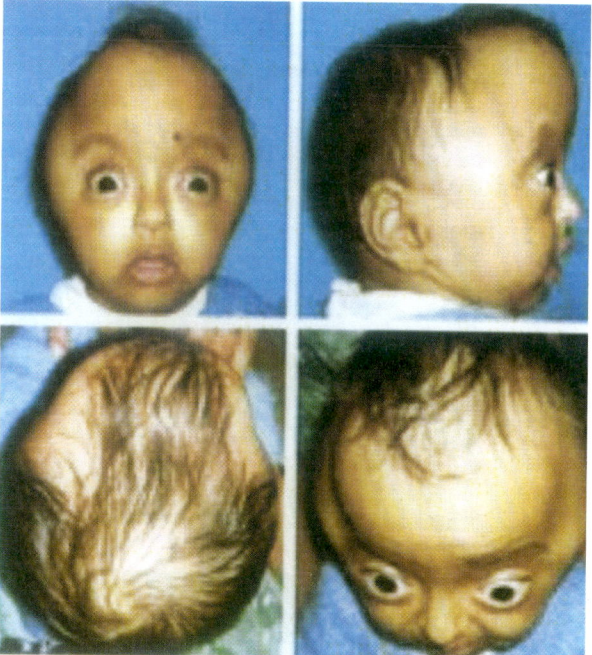

Fig. 10.12: Craniosynostosis

hypoplastic maxilla, short upper and protruding lower lips, hypertelorism and exophthalmos and external strabismus. Clover leaf skull syndrome (Kleeblattschadel), the X-ray skull in frontal view shows typical trilobed configuration. It is due to premature closure of some sutures and is associated with marked hydrocephalus, the skull bulges towards the temporal and frontal regions. It is often associated with other skeletal dysplasias.

Achondroplasia

It is the most common genetic skeletal dysplasia, transmitted as an autosomal dominant trait. Incidence is about 1 in 25,000 births, out of which 80% are new mutations. Clinical features of rhizomelic shortening of limbs (Fig. 10.13) present at birth is characteristic. The condition was so named by Parrot in 1878 as commonly used, than it is chondrodystrophia foetalis or micromelia. It is inherited as autosomal dominant gene, affecting the endochondral ossification.

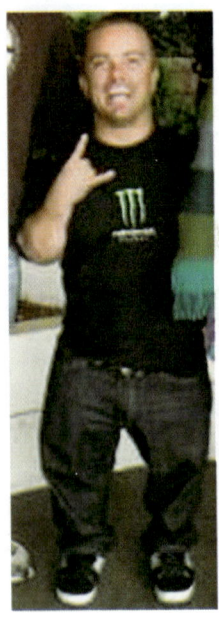

Fig. 10.13: Achondroplasia

The other clinical features are large head with frontal bossing, depression of nasal bridge, and short stature. The limbs are covered with fatty folds of skin in infancy and early childhood. The hands are short and broad. Lumbar gibbus is common in infancy but after first year this gibbus almost disappears and replaced by lumbar lordosis invariably.

Achondroplastic infants are often hypotonic with delayed motor development. Normal neuromuscular tone comes by the age of 2–3 years. Joint laxity particularly of the interphalangeal joints may persist throughout childhood. The head is large throughout life, with frontal bossing, hypoplasia of maxilla and relative mandibular prognathism. The intelligence, dentition and sexual development are normal, and musculature well developed so as to show surprising acrobatic feats. The pelvis is rotated forward giving rise to typical waddling gait with bowed legs.

Cleft Lip and Palate

The cleft lip and palate are distinct entities closely related embryologically, functionally and genetically. The cleft lip due to nonfusion of mesenchymal layers of maxillary and medial nasal processes, while cleft palate is due to non-fusion of palatal processes of maxillar arches and with the primitive palate (Fig. 10.14).

The incidence of cleft lip with or without cleft palate is 1 in 1000 births; the incidence of cleft palate alone is 1 in 2500 births. Sexual predominance of males is more in cleft lip with or without cleft palate as are the genetic factors than cleft palate alone. The risk of recurrence of cleft lip and palate is 4% for a couple, one affected child but increased to 9% if they had 2 affected children. The incidence of associated malformations specially of the structures derived from the first branchial arch, and intellectual impairment is increased in children with cleft palate alone. Clinically, the following combinations or forms are described.

1. Small notch in vermilion border to a complete separation extending into the nasal floor.

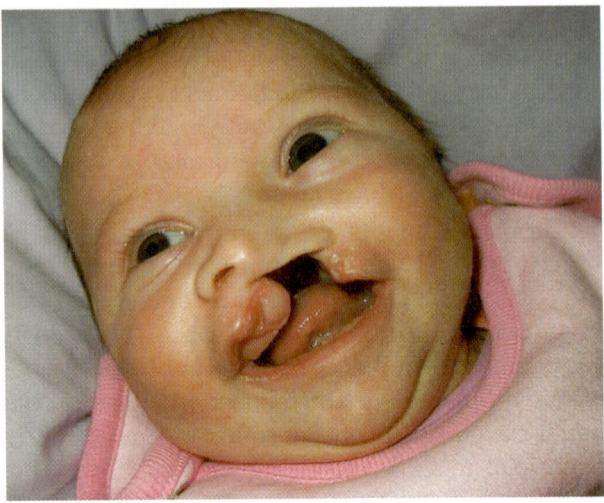

Fig. 10.14: Cleft lip and palate

2. Unilateral or bilateral clefts involving the alveolar ridge. Associated with deformed, supernumary or absent teeth.
3. The nasal cartilage clefts of lip, frequently associated with deficient columella, elongated vomer producing cleft premaxillary process.
4. A midline isolated cleft palate involving only uvula or extending upto incisive foramen.
5. When associated with cleft lip, the defect may involve the midline of soft palate and extend into the hard palate on one or both sides, exposing one or both of the nasal cavities as a unilateral or bilateral cleft palate. Pierre Robin Syndrome consists of micrognathia glossoptosis and high arched cleft palate.

Treacher Collins or Franceschetti syndrome (Mandibulo-facial dysostosis) consists of typical faces with sloping and downward palpebral fissures towards the outer cahthi, coloboma of lower eyelids, sunken cheek bones, blind fistulas opening between the angles of mouth and ears, deformed pinna, a typical hair growth extending towards cheek, receding chin and large mouth. Facial clefts, abnormalities of ears and deafness are common, autosomal dominant and incompletely expressed.

Hydrocephalus

This condition is due to enlargement of ventricles of brain resulting from imbalance between production and absorption of cerebrospinal-fluid, rarely due to overproduction of fluid. A number of congenital and acquired conditions lead to hydrocephalus (Fig. 10.15). Two anatomic types are distinguished.

   i. Obstructive hydrocephalus.

  ii. Communicating hydrocephalus.

Causes of obstruction can be congenital aqueductal stenosis or acquired due to infection, midline brain tumours, malformation of vein of galen, subdural haematoma in posterior cranial fossa and Dandy-Walker malformation.

In communicating type the interference with the absorption of CSF. Causes of obstruction in this type are also congenital as in Arnold–Chiari malformation, Hurler syndrome, achodroplasia and acquired like post-infectious meningitis, toxoplasmosis, cytomegalovirus infections, secondary to

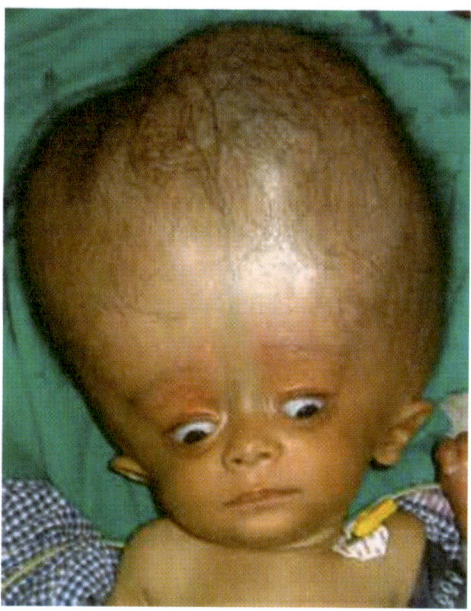

Fig. 10.15: Hydrocephalus

subarachnoid heamorrhage, papilloma of choroid plexus, vitamin A intoxication leading to excessive production of CSF.

Clinical features depend on time of onset and severity of imbalance between CSF production and resorption capacity. There is abnormal enlargement of head, even before birth causing difficulty during parturition, a common feature. In milder forms the head is normal at birth but grows at an excessive speed and serial measurements of head circumference are required for early diagnosis. The skull is distended in all directions but specially in frontal area. Occipital expansion is seen in Dandy Walker malformation as a result of dilation of fourth ventricle. A resonant sound on percussion of skull called *Macewen or cracked pot sign*, the scalp skin is thin and shiny with prominent scalp veins, the child has high pitched cry, eyes appear deviated downwards (setting sun sign) and optic atrophy may occur in untreated cases.

Phenylketonuria

This disorder occurs due to complete deficiency of phenylalinine hydroxylase enzyme.

The affected child is normal at birth but blonder than unaffected siblings. They have fair skin and blue eyes (Fig. 10.16), may have a seborrheic or eczematoid skin rash, which disappears as the child grows. Diagnosis depends on measuring blood levels of phenylalinine. The association of mental retardation with excretion of phenylpyruvic acid in urine was first noted in 1934 by Foling and in 1953 Bickel and Wolf suggested that this mental retardation can be prevented by giving diet low in phenylalinine and thus led to the first treatment for error of protein metabolism via diet. PKU is transmitted as an autosomal recessive disorder. The incidence is 1 in 20,000 caucasian births, but there is probably much geographic variation, though accurate data for other ethenic groups is lacking. Some heterozygotes may be identified by showing abnormally high blood levels of phenylalinine 1–4 hours after a loading dose (100 mg per kg). Maternal phenyla-linaemia may cause fetal brain damage with microcephaly and mental retardation in some cases, the mother being

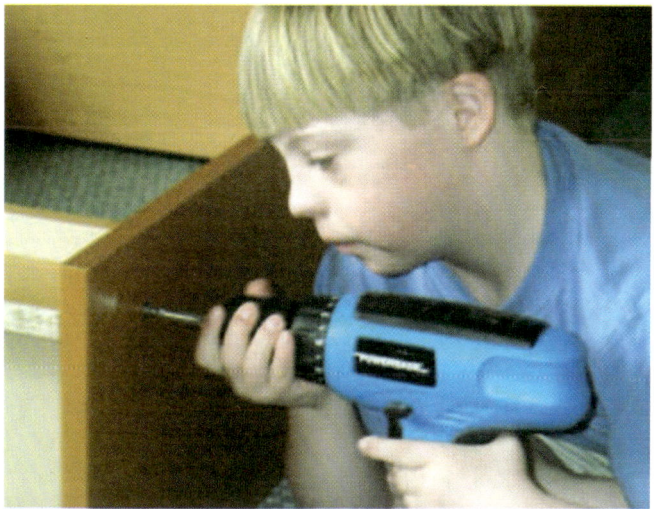

Fig. 10.16: Phenylketonuria

asymptomatic. Thus, routine screening for PKU in early pregnancy is logical though not yet practised. Intermediate forms of hyperphenylalaninemia noted during screening tests for PKU, showing blood levels of phenylalanine well below 1.2 mmol and brain damage does not occur. Some may show partial defect of hydroxylase enzyme, some may be heterozygote for PKU and some children may show transitory delay in enzyme maturation. Differentiation of these benign disorders from the classic PKU is sometimes difficult.

Cornelia de Lange Syndrome

This is one of the multiple malformation syndromes, with unknown aetiology and occurring as sporadic cases in otherwise normal families. The frequency is 1 in 10,300 cases. The characteristic features are Lobster claw hand (Fig. 10.17), associated with cleft lip and palate. Bushy eyebrows that almost meet in midline. Upper lips may be downturned.

Congenital Pigmented Nevi

Nevocellular nevi are present in about 1% of newborn infants, and pose more concern than the acquired ones because of

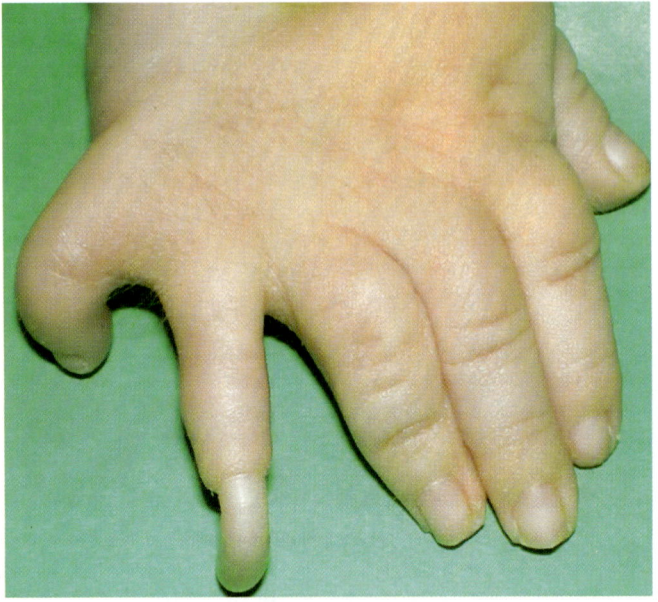

Fig. 10.17: Comelia de Lange syndrome

increased risk of development into malignant melanomas. Sites of predeliction are lower trunk and upper back, shoulders, proximal limbs and chest (Fig. 10.18). The lesions may be flat or elevated or nodular. They may appear in shades of brown, blue, or black and may develop numerous coarse hairs or remain hairless and leathery in texture. The term giant congenital pigmented nevi is used for nevi measuring < than 20 cm. Numerous smaller nevi may be scattered elsewhere. Giant pigmented nevi are of special significance for two reasons.

i. Its association with leptomeningeal melanocytosis.
ii. Predisposition for development of malignant melanoma. The involvement of leptomeninges may cause hydrocephalous seizures, retardation, motor deficit and may result in melartoma.

Persons with this disorder have spina bifida defect and pigmented rash all over the chest and hairy large pigmented areas on both thighs.

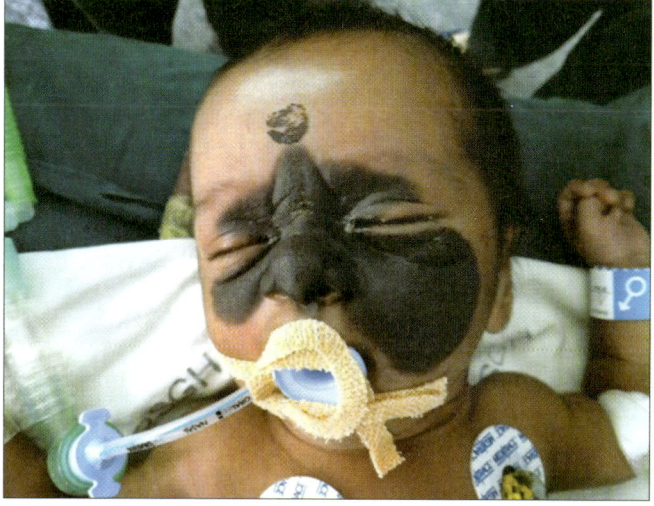

Fig. 10.18: Congenital pigmented nevi

Sacrococcygeal Teratoma

This is most common solid tumour in newborns (1 in 40,000 live births) with female preponderance. The most common finding is a mass in the region of sacrum and buttocks (Fig. 10.19). The incidence of malignancy is 10, if diagnosed at less than two months of age, and increases to 50 to 70% for tumours diagnosed after this age. Additional signs and symptoms depend on the growing tumur causing obstruction of rectum or urinary tract. Associated clinical features include congenital anomalies involving the lower vertebrae, genitourinary system or anorectal region. Other conditions of sacrococcygeal mass include meningoceles, chordomas, rhabdomyo-sarcomas, lipoma, and haemangioma. Sometimes masses in this area may be confused with perirectal abscess.

Anorectal Malformations

Congenital anamolies of anus and rectum are common, the incidence of minor abnormalities being 1,200 live births and major anamolies being 15,000 live births. Clinical classification of low and high types is in accordance with whether rectum

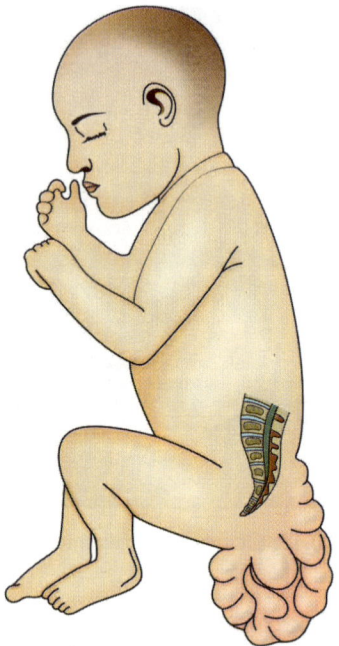

Fig. 10.19

does or does not pass through the puborectalis muscle—a major portion of levator ant muscle for defecation. Developmentally, the anus and rectum are derived from the dorsal part of cloaca after it is separated by a mesodermal urorectal septum in the midline, separating the ventral urinary bladder and urethra from dorsal rectum and anal canal. A small communication between the two systems, a cloacal duct is closed by 7th week of gestation. The urogenital portion of cloacal membrane ruptures by 7th week and anal portion ruptures by 8th week. Interference with the development of anorectal structures at varying stages gives rise to anomalies ranging from incomplete rupture of anal membrane or anal agenesis (the low type) (Fig. 10.20) to complete failure of descent of upper portion of cloaca and failure of invagination of proctodeum (the high type). Persistance of communication between urinary and rectal portions results in fistulas, more common in males. In females fistulas connect the rectum to vagina rather than urinar system.

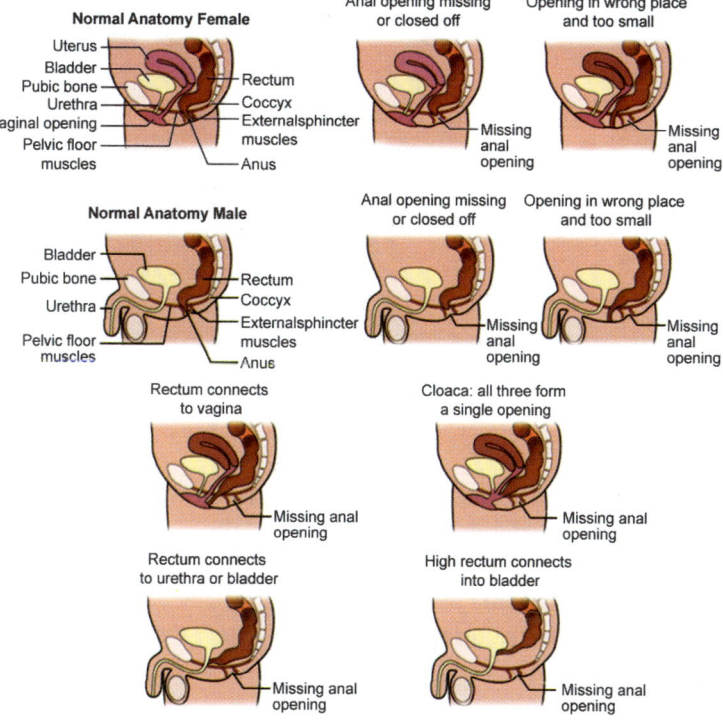

Fig. 10.20: Anorectal malformations

Cystic Hygroma (Lymphangioma)

Lymphangiomas are found in the region of neck or head in about 3/4 cases of benign tumours in children, appearing early in life by about three years of age. Some have been diagnosed antenatally during ultrasonic examination of mother (Fig. 10.21). The embryonic origin of lymphangiomas is uncertain, it can be a malformation, benign neoplasm, or a hamartoma. It may present as a unilocular or multicystic mass with thin and often transparent wall. The contents of the cysts are straw coloured. Cystic hygroma is compressible and cystic, non-tender or not painful. Ten per cent cases show intrathoracic extension, and the tumour may press on trachea leading to respiratory embarrassment. The tongue may also be involved and enlarged in some.

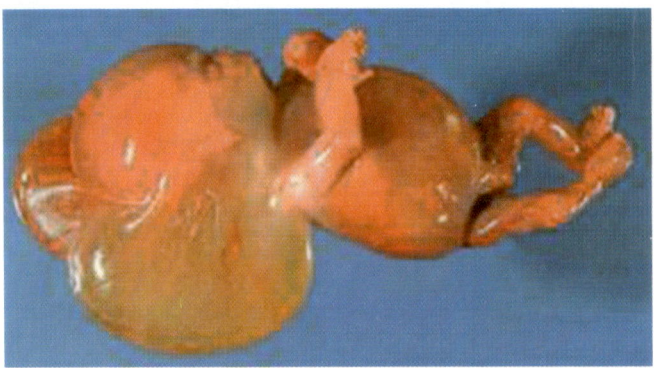

Fig. 10.21: Lymphangioma

EXERCISE

1. Enumerate patterns of single gene mutations.
2. Enumerate variants of trisomy syndrome.
3. Deficiency of 21-hydroxylase accounts for which congenital anomaly, exlplain.
4. What are the syndromes named due to defects in sex chromosomes?
5. Fill in the blanks.
    a. PKU stand for .... and is due to deficiency of ....
    b. Lobster claw hand is seen in ....
    c. Imperforate anus/anorectal malformation incidence is ....

Glossary

Agglutination: Cells joined together, or clumped, due to the action of antibody molecules.

Alleles (or allelomorphs): Genes which behave as alternatives in inheritance.

Amino acid: An organic compound containing both carboxyl ($-COOH$) and amino ($-NH_2$) groups.

Anaphase: The stage in mitosis (or meiosis II) in which longitudinal halves of metaphase chromosomes separate and migrate to opposite poles. During anaphase of the first meiotic division, homologous chromosomes in which crossing over has occurred segregate.

Aneuploid: Containing a chromosome number which is not an exact multiple of the haploid number, e.g. $2n - 1$ or $2n + 1$ where n is the haploid number of chromosomes.

Antenatal diagnosis: Determination of the genetical constitution of the phenotype of a foetus in utero. (Syn. prenatal diagnosis).

Antibody: A serum protein (immunoglobin) which is formed in response to an antigenic stimulus and reacts specifically with this antigen.

Antigen: A substance which elicits the synthesis of antibody with which it also reacts specifically.

Antigenic determinant: The part of an antigenic molecule against which the antibody is specifically directed.

Autoradiograph: Pattern of exposure of photographic film produced by radioactive decay, e.g. tritium incorporated into chromosomes as thymidine, which gives information regarding the incorporation of the radioactive precursor.

Autosome: Any chromosome other than the sex chromosomes. In men there are 22 pairs of autosomes.

Bacteriophage: A virus which infects bacteria.

Balanced polymorphism: A polymorphism at a locus maintained by selective advantage of the heterozygote over homozygotes.

Carrier: Heterozygote for a particular trait, usually recessive.

Cell cycle: The sequence of cellular events between two mitosis. It is customarily divided into four phases: mitosis synthetic or S-phase, when DNA is being replicated; Gl, the phase between mitosis and the S-phase; and G2, the phase between S and the next mitosis.

Centromere: The primary constriction of the chromosome, which becomes attached to the spindle during cell division. Sometimes called 'kinetochore'.

Chiasma: The cross configuration of chromatids of homologous chromo-somes during the first meiotic division, formed as a result of crossing over.

Chimera: An individual with genetically distinct cell lines originating from more than one zygote.

Chromatid: A longitudinal half of a chromosome during cell division before the division of the centromere in anaphase of mitosis or meiosis II.

Chromosomal aberration: An abnormality of chromosome number or structure.

Chromosomes: Thread-like, deep-staining bodies found within the nucleus. They are composed of DNA, RNA and protein and carry the genetical information. An acrocentric chromosome is one with the centromere located near the end of the chromosome, a metacentric chromosome is one with the centromere located near the middle of the chromosome.

Cistron: The functional unit of the hereditary material, as defined by the phenotype of a heterozygote carrying two recessive mutations from different parent; if the phenotype is a mutant, the genes concerned belong to the same cistron; if the phenotype is normal, the genes belong to different cistrons.

Codominance: When both alleles are expressed in the heterozygote.

Codon: A triplet of bases in the DNA or RNA molecule which codes for one aminoacid.

Complement: A system of nine serum protein components which act sequentially upon many antibody–antigen complexes, particularly when the antigen is cellular. The final effect of their sequential interaction is lysis with destruction of cellular antigens.

Congenital: Refers to any condition, whether genetically determined or not, which is present at birth.

Consanguineous marriage: A marriage between blood relatives, that is between persons who have one or more common ancestors.

Correlation: The corelationship of two variables. A correlation coefficient attempts to measure the interdependence of the two variables.

Cross over: The exchange of genetic material between homologous chromosomes at meiosis.

Cytogenetics: The branch of genetics concerned with the study of chromosomes and cellular phenomena.

Cytoplasm: The ground substance of the cell in which the nucleus, endoplasmic reticulum, mitochondria, etc. are present.

Deletion: The type of chromosomal aberration in which there is a loss of part of a chromosome (also called a deficiency).

Dermatoglyphics: The scientific study of the patterns of skin ridges on the fingers, toes, palms and soles.

Diakinesia: The last stage in the prophase of meiosis I, when the paired homologous chromosomes are highly contracted before they have moved onto the metaphase plate.

Diploid: The condition in which the cell contains two homologous sets of chromosomes. Normal state of somatic cells in mammals. Man's diploid number ($2n$) is 46.

Diplotene: The stage in the prophase of meiosis I, when the paired homologous chromosomes separate and are held together by chiasmata.

Dizygotic: Type of twins produced by the fertilization of two different ova by two different sperms. Dizygotic/fraternal/twins are no more similar genetically than are single brothers and sisters.

DNA (deoxyribonucleic acid): A polymer of nucleotides, where the pentose sugar (ribose) is in the deoxy form. DNA is found mainly in chromosomes but is present also in mitochondria. It represents the genetic material.

Dominant: A trait which is expressed in individuals who are heterozygous for a particular gene. Partial, incomplete, or semidominants are traits which are expressed in a reduced, incomplete or intermediate form in individuals who are heterozygous for a particular gene; many rare human dominants may be of this type, appropriate homozygotes not yet having been observed.

Drift: Random fluctuation in gene frequency in a population of finite size.

Duplication: A type of chromosomal aberration in which part of a chromosome is duplicated.

Euchromatin: The material basis of chromosomes and chromosomal regions which replicate their DNA early and exhibit other properties in contrast to heterochromatin.

Eugenics: The improvement of man by decreasing the frequency of definitely unfavourable genotypes (negative eugenics) and increasing the frequency of definitely favourable genotypes (positive eugenics).

Euploid: Containing either the haploid chromosome number or an exact multiple thereof.

Expressivity: Degree of severity of the expression of a particular gene.

Facultative heterochromatin: The material basis of chromosomes which exhibit heterochromatic properties only in the presence of an euchromatic partner, e.g. one X-chromosome in female mammals.

Gamete: A germ cell (sperm or ovum), normally containing a haploid number of chromosome.

Gene: The unit of inheritance, usually implying that section of a linkage group which behaves as a unit of function, i.e. the cistron. The commonest function is to code for a polypeptide chain.

Genetical counselling: The process of imparting advice to couples concerning the risks of handicap among their projected offspring and also concerning possibilities of circumventing these risks.

Genome: All the genetical material present in a typical cell of an organism.

Genotype: The genetical constitution of an individual.

Haploid: The condition in which the cell contains one set of chromosomes. Normal state of gametes in man where the haploid number is 23.

Hardy–Weinberg rule: An isolated population undergoing random mating in the absence of selection and mutation reaches genotypic equilibrium at an autosomal locus after one generation.

Hemizygous: The genotype of a male for an X-linked trait, since males have only one set of X-linked genes, or the genotype for loci on a monosomic autosome or loci on an autosome whose homologue bears an appropriate deletion.

Heritability: The proportion of the total variation of a character attributable to genetical as opposed to environmental factors.

Heterochromatin: The material basis of chromosomes or chromosomal regions which replicate their DNA late and frequently shows specific staining reactions. It is thought that heterochromatin is either devoid of genes or, if genes are present, they are not expressed (see also **constitutive, facultative heterochromatin**).

Heterogametic sex: The sex which produces gametes of two types with respect to the sex chromosomes. In man, the male is the heterogametic sex because he produces X-and Y-bearing sperms.

Heterozygote: An individual with two different alleles. (see also **Homozygote)**

Holandric inheritance: The pattern of inheritance of genes on to Y-chromosome. Only males are affected and the trait is transmitted by affected males to all their sons but to none of their daughters.

Homogametic sex: The sex which produces gametes of only one type with respect to the sex chromosomes. In humans, the female is the homogametic sex because she produces only X-bearing gametes.

Homologous chromosomes: Chromosomes derived from the father and mother respectively which pair during meiosis and contain identical loci.

Homozygote: An individual with two identical alleles.

Hybrid: The progeny of a cross between two genetically different organisms.

Immunodiffusion: A technique for the detection of specific antigens in solution by the reaction of antigen and antibody to form a precipitate in a gel medium.

Immunoglobulin: Inborn error of metabolism: A defect of intermediary metabolism which shows a Mendelian mode of inheritance, usually recessive (see also **Antibody**).

Inbreeding: The mating of individuals who are related by ancestry.

Inbreeding coefficient: The probability that the two genes at any locus in an individual are identical by descent, i.e., they originated from the replication of one gene in a previous generation.

Incidence: The frequency of occurrence of a trait or disease in a population, often over a specific interval of age or time.

Incompatibility: The situation when tissues from two antigenically distinct individuals are brought together, e.g. the relation between donor and host when a graft is rejected.

Interphase: The stage between two successive cell divisions during which DNA replication occurs.

Inversion: A type of chromosomal aberration in which two linear sequence of a chromosomal region is reversed.

Isoalleles: Functionally indistinguishable alleles at a locus.

Isochromosome: A type of chromosomal aberration in which one of the arms of a particular chromosome is duplicated and the other arm is deleted. The two arms of an isochromosome are therefore of equal length and contain the same genes.

Karyotype: The number, size and shape (and bands) of the chromosomes of a somatic cell. A photomicrograph of the chromosomes in one cell arranged in a standard manner, intended to be representative for the individual's a whole.

Kinetochote: see **Centromere**.

Linkage: Association on the same chromosome of two or more non-allelomorphic genes so that the combination of characters in offsprings tend to be different from that expected on the basis of independent assortment.

Locus: The position in a linkage map recognized as the site of an allelic difference.

Lyon hypothesis: The postulate that dosage compensation for genes on the X-chromosome in female eutherian mammals is achieved by the random permanent inactivation, at an early stage of embryogenesis of one or other of the X-chromosomes.

Meiosis: The type of cell division which occurs during gametogenesis and results in halving of the somatic number of chromosomes so that each gamete is haploid.

Metaphase: The stage of cell division when the contracted chromosomes line up on the equatorial plate, the nuclear membrane having disappeared.

Mitochondria: Subcellular organelles situated within the cytoplasm which are concerned with cellular respiration and oxidative phosphorylation.

Mitosis: The type of cell division which occurs in somatic cells maintaining a constant chromosome number.

Monosomy: Loss of one member of a chromosome pair so that there is one less than the diploid number of chromosomes ($2n - 1$).

Monozygotic: Type of twin pair derived from a single fertilized ovum, also called identical.

Mosaic: An individual with genetically distinct cell lines originating from a single zygote.

Multifactorial: Determination by many genes with small effects together with the effects of the environment.

Multiple alleles: The existence of more than two alleles for a particular character.

Mutation: A change in the genetical material, either of a single gene (point mutation) or in the number or structure of the chromosomes. A mutation which occurs in the gametes (germinal) is inherited, a mutation which occurs in the somatic cells (somatic mutation) is not inherited.

Mutation rates: The number of mutations of any one particular unit of inheritance (cistron, gene, etc.) which occur per gamete per generation.

Non-dysjunction: The failure of two members of a chromosome pair to separate during cell division. This means that both pass to the same daughter cell.

Non-homologous cross over: Exchange of nonhomologous segments of chromosomes at meiosis. This event results in reciprocal deletion and duplication of the involved chromosome segments.

Normal distribution (Gaussian distribution): A continuous symmetrical bell-shaped distribution, usually plotting the frequency of observations.

Nucleous: A spheroidal structure within the nucleus, which occurs in association with a particular locus (the nucleolar organizer) on a specific chromosome.

Nucleotide: Nucleic acids are made up of sequences of many nucleotides each of which consists of a nitrogenous base, a pentose sugar, and a phosphate group.

Nucleus: A structure within the cell which contains the chromosomes and nucleus.

Operator: The binding site for a represser molecule, at one end of an operon.

Operon: A group of closely linked genes in bacteria which apparently affect different steps in a particular metabolic pathway and which seem to function as an integrated unit.

Overdominance: Heterozygous advantage at a locus with two alleles the heterozygote is fitter than either homozygote, giving rise to a balanced polymorphism.

Pachytene: The stage in the prophase of meiosis I, when the fully paired homologous chromosomes are partially contracted.

Penetrance: Proportion of a genotype manifesting a trait. If some with the genotype do not manifest the trait, there is reduced penetrance.

Pharmacogenetics: The study of genetically determined variations in individual response to drug therapy.

Phenocopy: A condition which is due to environmental factors but resembles one which is genetically determined.

Phenotype: The appearance (with respect to some physical, biochemical, physiological characters of an individual which results from the interaction of genotype and environment.

Pleiotropy: A gene with multiple effects is said to be pleiotropic.

Polygenic: Inheritance controlled by many genes each having a small effect.

Polymorphism: The occurrence in a population of two or more genetically determined forms in such frequencies that the rarest of them could not be maintained by mutation alone. The alleles determining such forms are known as polymorphic alleles or polymorphs (see also **balanced polymorphism, transient polymorphism**).

Polypeptide: An organic compound consisting of three or more aminoacids which are linked covalently through amide bonds, the functional product of the translation of messenger RNA.

Polyploid: Having any multiple greater than two of the haploid number of chromosomes, e.g. $3n$, $4n$, etc.

Prevalence: The observed frequency of a trait or disease in a population, often at a particular age or time.

Proband (or index case): An affected individual (irrespective of sex) through whom the family came to the attention of the investigator.

Propositus *if a male;* **proposita** *if a female.*

Pro-metaphase: The stage in mitosis between the dissolution of the nuclear membrane and the organization of the chromosome on the metaphase plate.

Prophase: The first visible stage of cell division when the chromosomes are contracted and, therefore, thicker, but before breakdown of the nuclear membranes.

Protein: A complex organic polypeptide macromolecule with enzymatic, structural, or transport function.

Random gentical drift: See *drift*.

Random mating: Selection of a spouse without regard for the spouse's genotype.

Recessive: A trait expressed in individuals who are homozygous for a particular gene but not in those who are heterozygous for this gene.

Recombination: The process whereby new combinations of parental characters may arise in the progeny. The term recombinant chromosome is used for one which is present in the haploid set of the gamete and which because of crossing over, at meiosis contains a combination of genes distinct from that found on either of the parental homologues from which it is derived.

Regulator gene: A gene which synthesizes a represser substance which inhibits the action of a specific operon, according to the Jacob and Monod theory. In a more general way, a regulatory gene is any which influences the expression of a *structural gene*, e.g. by controlling enzyme activity, enzyme synthesis or enzyme breakdown.

Ribosomes: Subcellular organelles situated in the cytoplasm, which are associated with protein synthesis. In mammalian cells, ribosomes are attached to the endoplasmic reticulum.

RNA (ribonucleic acid): The nucleic acid which is found mainly in the nucleus and ribosomes. *Messenger-RNA* transfers genetic information from the nucleus to the ribosomes in the cytoplasm and also acts as a template for the synthesis of polypeptides. *Transfer-RNA* transfers activated aminoacids from the cytoplasm to messenger-RNA.

Segregation: The separation of alleles during meiosis so that each gamete contains only one member of each pair of alleles.

Selection: The forces which affect biological fitness and, therefore, the frequency of a particular condition within a given population.

Sex chromatin: A body constituting a sex chromosome, or part there of which is visible in an interphase nucleus (1) Barr body—darkly stained mass," usually situated at the periphery of an interphase nucleus in cells" contains two X-chromosomes (or more), representing one of the X-chromosomes in a condensed and inactive form. (2) Drumstick—special nuclear appendage present in a proportion of polymorpho-nucleaf leucocytes containing two X-chromosomes (or more). (3) Fluorescent Y-body—fluorescent body visible in interphase cells containing a Y-chromosome.

Sex chromosomes: The chromosomes which differ in males and females (XX in women, XY in men) and which are responsible for sex determination.

Sex linkage: Genes carried on the sex chromosomes. Since there are very few Mendelian genes on the Y-chromosome, if any, the term is often used synonymously with X-linkage.

Sib (or sibling): Brother or sister.

Spindle: A structure responsible for the movement of the chromosomes during cell division.

Structural gene: One whose base sequence determines the primary structure of its product. If the product is a polypeptide, the primary structure will be its amino acid sequence; if it is a ribosomal or a transfer RNA, its primary structure will be the sequence of its purine and pyrimidine bases.

Syndrome: A characteristic constellation of anomalies and/or symptoms which consistently occur together in individuals.

Syntenic: Of loci in the same linkage group and thus on the same chromosome.

Telophase: The stage of cell division when the chromosomes have completely separated into two groups and each group has become invested in a nuclear membrane.

Threshold: A critical value on an underlying scale of liability above which individuals manifest a trait or disease. See also **Liability.**

Transcription: The process whereby genetic information is Transmitted from the DNA in the chromosomes to messenger-RNA.

Translation: The process whereby genetic information from messenger-RNA is translated into protein synthesis.

Translocation: The transfer part of one chromosome to another non-homologous chromosome. If there is an exchange of parts between two chromosomes, this is referred to as a reciprocal translocation. The term translocation also refers to a detailed step in biosynthesis of polypeptide chain

Triplet: A series of three bases in the DNA or RNA molecule which codes for a specific amino acid.

Triploid: A cell with three haploid sets of chromosomes, i.e. $3n$.

Trisomy: Presence of one chromosome in triplicate instead of in duplicate.

Unifactorial: Inheritance controlled by a single gene pair.

X-linkage: Genes carried on the X-chromosome are said to be X-linked.

Zygote: The fertilized ovum.

Zygotene: The stage of meiosis (part of prophase I) when the homologous chromosmes are side by side.

Index